T0239982

OTHER FAST FACTS BOOKS

Fast Facts on **ADOLESCENT HEALTH FOR NURSING AND HEALTH PROFESSIONALS**: A Care Guide *(Herrman)*

Fast Facts for the **ANTEPARTUM AND POSTPARTUM NURSE**: A Nursing Orientation and Care Guide *(Davidson)*

Fast Facts Workbook for **CARDIAC DYSRHYTHMIAS AND 12-LEAD EKGs** *(Desmarais)*

Fast Facts for the **CARDIAC SURGERY NURSE**: Caring for Cardiac Surgery Patients, Third Edition *(Hodge)*

Fast Facts for **CAREER SUCCESS IN NURSING**: Making the Most of Mentoring *(Vance)*

Fast Facts for the **CATH LAB NURSE** *(McCulloch)*

Fast Facts for the **CLASSROOM NURSING INSTRUCTOR**: Classroom Teaching *(Yoder-Wise, Kowalski)*

Fast Facts for the **CLINICAL NURSE LEADER** *(Wilcox, Deerhake)*

Fast Facts for the **CLINICAL NURSE MANAGER**: Managing a Changing Workplace, Second Edition *(Fry)*

Fast Facts for the **CLINICAL NURSING INSTRUCTOR**: Clinical Teaching, Third Edition *(Kan, Stabler-Haas)*

Fast Facts on **COMBATING NURSE BULLYING, INCIVILITY, AND WORKPLACE VIOLENCE**: What Nurses Need to Know *(Ciocco)*

Fast Facts for the **CRITICAL CARE NURSE**, Second Edition *(Hewett)*

Fast Facts About **CURRICULUM DEVELOPMENT IN NURSING**: How to Develop and Evaluate Educational Programs, Second Edition *(McCoy, Anema)*

Fast Facts for **DEMENTIA CARE**: What Nurses Need to Know, Second Edition *(Miller)*

Fast Facts for **DEVELOPING A NURSING ACADEMIC PORTFOLIO**: What You Really Need to Know *(Wittmann-Price)*

Fast Facts for **DNP ROLE DEVELOPMENT**: A Career Navigation Guide *(Menonna-Quinn, Tortorella Genova)*

Fast Facts About **EKGs FOR NURSES**: The Rules of Identifying EKGs *(Landrum)*

Fast Facts for the **ER NURSE**: Emergency Department Orientation, Third Edition *(Buettner)*

Fast Facts for **EVIDENCE-BASED PRACTICE IN NURSING**: Third Edition *(Godshall)*

Fast Facts for the **FAITH COMMUNITY NURSE**: Implementing FCN/Parish Nursing *(Hickman)*

Fast Facts About **FORENSIC NURSING**: What You Need to Know *(Scannell)*

Fast Facts for the **GERONTOLOGY NURSE**: A Nursing Care Guide *(Eliopoulos)*

Fast Facts About **GI AND LIVER DISEASES FOR NURSES**: What APRNs Need to Know *(Chaney)*

Fast Facts About the **GYNECOLOGICAL EXAM**: A Professional Guide for NPs, PAs, and Midwives, Second Edition *(Secor, Fantasia)*

Fast Facts in **HEALTH INFORMATICS FOR NURSES** *(Hardy)*

Fast Facts for **HEALTH PROMOTION IN NURSING**: Promoting Wellness *(Miller)*

Fast Facts for Nurses About **HOME INFUSION THERAPY**: The Expert's Best Practice Guide *(Gorski)*

Fast Facts for the **HOSPICE NURSE**: A Concise Guide to End-of-Life Care, Second Edition *(Wright)*

Fast Facts for the **L&D NURSE**: Labor & Delivery Orientation, Second Edition *(Groll)*

Fast Facts for the **LONG-TERM CARE NURSE**: What Nursing Home and Assisted Living Nurses Need to Know *(Eliopoulos)*

Fast Facts to **LOVING YOUR RESEARCH PROJECT**: A Stress-Free Guide for Novice Researchers in Nursing and Healthcare *(Marshall)*

Fast Facts for **MAKING THE MOST OF YOUR CAREER IN NURSING** *(Redulla)*

Fast Facts for **MANAGING PATIENTS WITH A PSYCHIATRIC DISORDER**: What RNs, NPs, and New Psych Nurses Need to Know *(Marshall)*

Fast Facts About **MEDICAL CANNABIS AND OPIOIDS**: Minimizing Opioid Use Through Cannabis *(Smith, Smith)*

Fast Facts for the **MEDICAL OFFICE NURSE**: What You Really Need to Know *(Richmeier)*

Fast Facts for the **MEDICAL–SURGICAL NURSE**: Clinical Orientation *(Ciocco)*

Fast Facts for the **NEONATAL NURSE**: A Nursing Orientation and Care Guide *(Davidson)*

Fast Facts About **NEUROCRITICAL CARE**: A Quick Reference for the Advanced Practice Provider *(McLaughlin)*

Fast Facts for the **NEW NURSE PRACTITIONER**: What You Really Need to Know, Second Edition *(Aktan)*

Fast Facts for **NURSE PRACTITIONERS:** Practice Essentials for Clinical Subspecialties *(Aktan)*

Fast Facts for the **NURSE PRECEPTOR**: Keys to Providing a Successful Preceptorship *(Ciocco)*

Fast Facts for the **NURSE PSYCHOTHERAPIST**: The Process of Becoming *(Jones, Tusaie)*

Fast Facts About **NURSING AND THE LAW**: Law for Nurses *(Grant, Ballard)*

Fast Facts About the **NURSING PROFESSION**: Historical Perspectives *(Hunt)*

Fast Facts for the **OPERATING ROOM NURSE**: An Orientation and Care Guide, Second Edition *(Criscitelli)*

Fast Facts for the **PEDIATRIC NURSE**: An Orientation Guide *(Rupert, Young)*

Fast Facts Handbook for **PEDIATRIC PRIMARY CARE:** A Guide for Nurse Practitioners and Physician Assistants *(Ruggiero, Ruggiero)*

Fast Facts About **PRESSURE ULCER CARE FOR NURSES**: How to Prevent, Detect, and Resolve Them *(Dziedzic)*

Fast Facts About **PTSD**: A Guide for Nurses and Other Health Care Professionals *(Adams)*

Fast Facts for the **RADIOLOGY NURSE**: An Orientation and Nursing Care Guide, Second Edition *(Grossman)*

Fast Facts About **RELIGION FOR NURSES**: Implications for Patient Care *(Taylor)*

Fast Facts for the **SCHOOL NURSE**: What You Need to Know, Third Edition *(Loschiavo)*

Fast Facts About **SEXUALLY TRANSMITTED INFECTIONS**: A Nurse's Guide to Expert Patient Care *(Scannell)*

Fast Facts for **STROKE CARE NURSING**: An Expert Care Guide, Second Edition *(Morrison)*

Fast Facts for the **STUDENT NURSE**: Nursing Student Success *(Stabler-Haas)*

Fast Facts About **SUBSTANCE USE DISORDERS**: What Every Nurse, APRN, and PA Needs to Know *(Marshall, Spencer)*

Fast Facts for the **TRAVEL NURSE**: Travel Nursing *(Landrum)*

Fast Facts for the **TRIAGE NURSE**: An Orientation and Care Guide, Second Edition *(Visser, Montejano)*

Fast Facts for the **WOUND CARE NURSE**: Practical Wound Management *(Kifer)*

Fast Facts for **WRITING THE DNP PROJECT**: Effective Structure, Content, and Presentation *(Christenbery)*

Forthcoming FAST FACTS Books

Fast Facts for the **ADULT-GERONTOLOGY ACUTE CARE NURSE PRACTITIONER** *(Carpenter)*

Fast Facts About **COMPETENCY-BASED EDUCATION IN NURSING**: How to Teach Competency Mastery *(Wittmann-Price, Gittings)*

Fast Facts for **CREATING A SUCCESSFUL TELEHEALTH SERVICE**: A How-to Guide for Nurse Practitioners *(Heidesch)*

Fast Facts About **DIVERSITY, EQUITY, AND INCLUSION** *(Davis)*

Fast Facts for the **ER NURSE**: Guide to a Successful Emergency Department Orientation, Fourth Edition *(Buettner)*

Fast Facts for the **L&D NURSE**: Labor & Delivery Orientation, Third Edition *(Groll)*

Fast Facts About **LGBTQ CARE FOR NURSES** *(Traister)*

Fast Facts for the **NEONATAL NURSE**: Care Essentials for Normal and High-Risk Neonates, Second Edition *(Davidson)*

Fast Facts for the **NURSE PRECEPTOR**: Keys to Providing a Successful Preceptorship, Second Edition *(Ciocco)*

Fast Facts for **PATIENT SAFETY IN NURSING** *(Hunt)*

Visit www.springerpub.com to order.

FAST FACTS for
NURSE PRACTITIONERS

Nadine M. Aktan, PhD, APN-BC, received her bachelor's, master's, and doctoral degrees in nursing from Rutgers University College of Nursing and Graduate School in New Brunswick and Newark, New Jersey. Having served as the chairperson of nursing at William Paterson University in Wayne, New Jersey, Dr. Aktan is currently professor of nursing focusing on teaching community health to future nurses and adult health and family practice to nurse practitioner students. She also practices as a family nurse practitioner at the Immedicenter, a primary care/urgent care/family practice with locations in Clifton, Bloomfield, and Totowa, New Jersey, and as a maternal–child and adult community health nurse for Valley Home Care in Paramus, New Jersey.

FAST FACTS for
NURSE PRACTITIONERS

Practice Essentials
for Clinical Subspecialties

Nadine M. Aktan, PhD, APN-BC

SPRINGER PUBLISHING COMPANY

Springer Publishing Company, LLC
11 West 42nd Street, New York, NY 10036
www.springerpub.com
connect.springerpub.com/

Acquisitions Editor: Jaclyn Koshofer
Compositor: Amnet Systems

ISBN: 978-0-8261-4872-8
ebook ISBN: 978-0-8261-4873-5
DOI: 10.1891/9780826148735

20 21 22 23 / 5 4 3 2 1

The author and the publisher of this Work have made every effort to use sources believed to be reliable to provide information that is accurate and compatible with the standards generally accepted at the time of publication. Because medical science is continually advancing, our knowledge base continues to expand. Therefore, as new information becomes available, changes in procedures become necessary. We recommend that the reader always consult current research and specific institutional policies before performing any clinical procedure or delivering any medication. The author and publisher shall not be liable for any special, consequential, or exemplary damages resulting, in whole or in part, from the readers' use of, or reliance on, the information contained in this book. The publisher has no responsibility for the persistence or accuracy of URLs for external or third-party Internet websites referred to in this publication and does not guarantee that any content on such websites is, or will remain, accurate or appropriate.

Library of Congress Cataloging-in-Publication Data
Names: Aktan, Nadine M., author.
Title: Fast facts for nurse practitioners : practice essentials for
    clinical subspecialties / Nadine M. Aktan.
Other titles: Fast facts (Springer Publishing Company)
Description: New York, NY : Springer Publishing Company, LLC, [2021] |
    Series: Fast facts | Includes bibliographical references and index.
Identifiers: LCCN 2020013664 (print) | LCCN 2020013665 (ebook) | ISBN
    9780826148728 (paperback) | ISBN 9780826148735 (ebook)
Subjects: MESH: Advanced Practice Nursing—methods | Nurse Practitioners |
    Nursing Care | Specialties, Nursing
Classification: LCC RT82.8 (print) | LCC RT82.8 (ebook) | NLM WY 128 |
    DDC 610.7306/92—dc23
LC record available at https://lccn.loc.gov/2020013664
LC ebook record available at https://lccn.loc.gov/2020013665

Contact us to receive discount rates on bulk purchases.
We can also customize our books to meet your needs.
For more information, please contact sales@springerpub.com.

Publisher's Note: New and used products purchased from third-party sellers are not guaranteed for quality, authenticity, or access to any included digital components.

Printed in the United States of America.

Contents

Preface

Fast Facts for Nurse Practitioners: Practice Essentials for Clinical Subspecialties initially explores how the role of the nurse practitioner has evolved and will continue to play an essential role in shaping healthcare—both today and in the future. Nursing has been long referred to as both an art and a science. It is a practice discipline. APRNs typically maintain competency by obtaining certifications, attending conferences, reading journals, and completing continuing education activities. As I approached my 20th year in advanced nursing practice, I decided to immerse myself in concentrated, clinical practice time with physicians and advanced practice nursing specialists. The aim of this project was to describe what was learned and provide the reader with the current standards of practice in the evaluation and management of conditions typically presented in primary care settings.

This book will stimulate both critical thinking and clinical reasoning. It will serve as a resource to advanced practice nursing students as well as practicing nurse practitioners. Each chapter presents a different clinical specialty area. Common primary care conditions are described with corresponding management plans. Although scientific and evidence based, the format is presented to the reader as part of the journey, making the book more desirable to the reader than the traditional textbook.

Global, complex health challenges must be solved in interdisciplinary, collaborative ways. APRNs work alongside all members of the healthcare team meaningfully and effectively. The goal of this book is for a seasoned nurse practitioner to share practical guidance, which supports the reader to be better prepared in the provision of high-quality primary care to their clients and families.

Nadine M. Aktan

Acknowledgments

Life is a series of adventures. I am grateful that my journey is one that has allowed me to touch the lives of others in positive ways throughout my nursing career. Although challenging at times, being a nurse, nurse practitioner, and academic nurse has led to some of my greatest professional achievements. I am forever thankful to my mentors in the disciplines of nursing, medicine, and academia for sharing their wisdom and passion. Specifically, for this project, I would like to acknowledge William Paterson University for awarding me the sabbatical, which allowed me the freedom to embark on this experience as well as select colleagues who welcomed me as I immersed myself in their clinical practice:

Melissa Algieri, MSN, APN-BC
Dr. Natalia Anchipolovsky
Dr. Sameer Azhak
Dr. Zamir Brelvi
Darlene Clemente, MSN, APN-BC
Dr. Lesley Fein
Dr. Ayal Kaynan
Dr. Ahuja Kishore
Joann Lane, MSN, APN-BC
Dr. Nidal Matalkah
Dr. Alan Miller
Dr. Meredith Schade

Thank you to my team of family and friends who have supported me in accomplishing my dreams. To my greatest advocate, my mother, Barbara, my partner in life, Mukbil, and my cherished gifts, my daughter, Delila, and my son, Jett. It takes a village, and I am lucky to have this network of love and strength behind me.

1

Advanced Practice Providers in Primary Care: Past and Present

The average annual healthcare costs in the United States were $24.7 billion in 1960 and estimated to be over $3,504 trillion in 2019. More and more Americans are going overseas for medical care and affordable prescription drugs. By 2030, the shortage of physicians will be between 40,000 and 120,000 (Association of American Medical Colleges, 2019), and artificial intelligence will begin to revolutionize healthcare. Currently, there are 270,000 nurse practitioners licensed to practice in the United States, and 25 states allow APRNs full practice authority (American Association of Nurse Practitioners, n.d.). Studies have found no significant differences in the quality of care that APRNs provide, such as prescribing habits, ordering of imaging studies, hospitalizations, readmissions, or emergency visits, as compared with our physician colleagues. Patient satisfaction has been reported to be higher in some studies, and in the management of primary care services, APRNs represented a cost savings of 11% to 29% (McCleery, Christensen, Peterson, Humphrey, & Helfand, 2014).

THE PAST

A social phenomenon occurred in the United States in the late 1950s and the early 1960s. There were shortages of pediatricians and family practice physicians, a lack of primary healthcare in rural areas, and limited access to healthcare services by the urban poor. These experiences lead to a collaboration between a pioneer nurse, Dr. Loretta Ford, and pediatrician, Dr. Henry Silver, to establish the first nurse practitioner program in 1965 at the University of Colorado (Ford, 1979).

Ford (1979) reported changing patterns in healthcare were occurring, which affected the role the professional nurses played in the delivery of care. Examples included soaring healthcare costs (8% of the gross national product in the United States), child abuse, health disparities, and occupational health risks. In the 1960s, there were also changes in values and questions being raised as to who had a right to health and healthcare. Healthcare was growing without a national policy. There was an increase in knowledge, cost, specialization, technology, demand, and complexity, all while a decrease of personnel was occurring. This resulted in a direct decrease in quality and distribution of services (Ford, 1979).

Ford (1979) also described issues with access to care and a fragmentation of services provided, which resulted in challenges in the coordination, continuity, quality, distribution, and financing of healthcare. There was an imbalance between curable and preventative care, which called for reorganizational designs in healthcare delivery with a focus on competition or choice for the consumer. Because America was failing at achieving significant improvements in healthcare quality, availability, and equity, new approaches to care had to be considered (e.g., priority setting, resource allocation, productivity evaluation) without expanding expenditure (Ford, 1979).

Ford (1979) noted a lack of incentives for providers in prevention, calling for a slowing down of technology in favor of health promotion and disease prevention. She advocated for rewards in reimbursement to be provided to physicians for surgical procedures, hospitalization, and episodic care. Disease-oriented medical services were also a point of discussion, as Ford noted a need for transitioning to aholistic, health-oriented care system where decisions on allocations of healthcare resources would be guided by a national health policy (Ford, 1979). According to Ford (1979), primary care services needed to focus on both the sick and the well to encompass both preventive and restorative care, health maintenance, and health education. She called for open access to care, continuity, and coordination, holding providers accountable for quality of care.

At this time, nursing, the largest single group of available healthcare workers, was moving from a technical occupation to a profession with a focus on commitment to care, advancing science, and increased accountability in decision-making. Ford (1979) shared that nurses were underutilized, underestimated, and undercompensated, as their scope of practice was continually expanding. In 1965, this led to the evolution of the role when the pediatric nurse practitioner, an expert in the provision of physical and psychological care to children in community settings, was developed. Pediatric histories, comprehensive exams, growth and development screenings, and management decisions of common childhood problems with an emphasis on well care and education of parents were provided (Ford, 1979).

Team care and joint practice were common developing patterns at this time. These models of practice were economical, as the nurses' skills are fully used and higher-priced physician services are provided only when necessary. The outcome was the effective utilization of clinical skills of professional nurses to increase quality of care, particularly in rural and urban areas where improved access was needed. There was also evidence of a greater confidence and professional satisfaction of the nursing workforce (Ford, 1979).

THE PRESENT

Many of the issues described by Ford remain prevalent today. In fact, healthcare spending grew 4.6% in 2018, reaching $3.6 trillion, accounting for 17.7% of our nation's gross domestic product (as compared with 8% in the 1960s; U.S. Centers for Medicare & Medicaid Services, n.d.). The role of nurses and APRNs has and must continue to evolve in accordance with these societal and economic influences. Currently, the master's degree is the minimal educational requirement of the APRN. The essentials of the master's education in nursing guide the preparation of advanced nursing graduates for diverse areas of practice in any healthcare setting. They are listed in Box 1.1.

Therefore, the APRNs of today are educated on many of the same fundamental concepts described by Dr. Ford such as nursing leadership in healthcare evolution, a greater emphasis on the quality of care provided and need for health promotion/disease prevention, the importance of incorporating evidence into practice, the role of technology in advancing care, the need for policy to allocate funds and guide practice, and the advancement of the nursing profession through collaboration and education.

In 2010, the Patient Protection and Affordable Care Act was enacted. The Supreme Court upheld its legality in 2012, making coverage for all Americans available at a cost through a variety of plans and company options. The legislation, however, has since evolved and the penalties for participation were waived in 2019. It has been reported that nursing professionals face challenges related to education and training, as well as a need for a clearer definition of nursing's role in primary healthcare. Furthermore, as a professional, they must overcome a number of difficulties such as fragmented care and invest in multidisciplinary teamwork, community empowerment,

BOX 1.1 AMERICAN ASSOCIATION OF COLLEGES OF NURSING'S ESSENTIALS OF MASTER'S EDUCATION IN NURSING

I.	Background for Practice from Sciences and Humanities
II.	Organizational and Systems Leadership
III.	Quality Improvement and Safety
IV.	Translating and Integrating Scholarship into Practice
V.	Informatics and Healthcare Technologies
VI.	Health Policy and Advocacy
VII.	Interprofessional Collaboration for Improving Patient and Population Health Outcomes
VIII.	Clinical Prevention and Population Health for Improving Health
IX.	Master's-Level Nursing Practice

Source: Data from American Association of Colleges of Nursing. (2011). The essentials of master's education in nursing. Retrieved from http://www .aacnnursing.org/portals/42/publications/mastersessentials11.pdf

professional–patient bond, user embracement, and soft technologies to promote quality of life, holistic care, and universal health coverage (Schveitzer, Zoboli, & Vieira, 2016).

THE FUTURE

To date, the DNP is not a requirement for advanced practice nursing licensure and certification. However, many APRNs have decided to advance their nursing education to the highest level, that is, the doctoral level. This degree promotes nursing to "sit at the table," so to speak with other colleagues in disciplines such as medicine, pharmacy, physical therapy, and psychology, where important decisions are made that promote positive healthcare outcomes both today and in the future. The DNP-prepared nursing professional works collaboratively with PhD-prepared nurses, experts in the collection, analysis, and dissemination of nursing research, and EdD-prepared nurses, experts in the design, implementation, and evaluation of nursing education. The DNP curriculum is not an add-on to the master's curriculum; instead, this curriculum integrates objectives

BOX 1.2 AMERICAN ASSOCIATION OF COLLEGES OF NURSING'S ESSENTIALS OF DOCTORAL EDUCATION FOR ADVANCED NURSING PRACTICE

I.	Scientific Underpinnings for Practice
II.	Organizational and Systems Leadership for Quality Improvement and Systems Thinking
III.	Clinical Scholarship and Analytical Methods for Evidence-Based Practice
IV.	Information Systems/Technology and Patient Care Technology for the Improvement and Transformation of Healthcare
V.	Healthcare Policy for Advocacy in Healthcare
VI.	Interprofessional Collaboration for Improving Patient and Population Health Outcomes
VII.	Clinical Prevention and Population Health for Improving the Nation's Health
VIII.	Advanced Nursing Practice

Source: Data from American Association of Colleges of Nursing. (2006). *The essentials of doctoral education for advanced nursing practice*. Retrieved from https://www.aacnnursing.org/Portals/42/Publications/DNPEssentials.pdf

and learning opportunities for students to achieve the core and population-focused competencies that are written for doctoral-level education (National Organization of Nurse Practitioner Faculties, 2018). The essentials for advanced nursing practice that guide the clinical education of nurses at the doctoral level are listed in Box 1.2.

The National Organization of Nurse Practitioner Faculties (NONPF, 2018) has committed to the movement of all entry-level nurse practitioner education to the DNP degree by 2025. It has been reported that, in 2018, there were more than 300 DNP programs throughout the United States. The NONPF leads the evolution of nurse practitioner education preparation to the doctoral level. The NONPF is dedicated to all currently credentialed nurse practitioners and faculty members; however, the group strongly recognizes that as the role has evolved, the healthcare delivery system has grown increasingly complex. The DNP degree reflects the rigorous education that nurse practitioners receive to lead and deliver quality healthcare (National Organization of Nurse Practitioner Faculties, 2018).

Fast Facts

- The evolution of the role of nursing to the advanced practice level has resulted in a greater confidence and professional satisfaction of the nursing workforce.
- Healthcare expenditure grew 4.6% in 2018, reaching $3.6 trillion, accounting for 17.7% of our nation's gross domestic product (as compared with 8% in the 1960s).
- The NONPF (2018) has committed to the movement of all entry-level nurse practitioner education to the DNP degree by 2025.
- The DNP degree reflects the rigorous education that nurse practitioners receive to lead and deliver quality healthcare.

SUMMARY

Nurse practitioners have been providing comprehensive, high-quality, evidence-based healthcare services to patients of all ages for more than a half century. As the nation's healthcare system continues to face increased morbidity and mortality and an array of fiscal challenges, coupled with provider shortages, there will be an increased demand for nurse practitioners to collaborate with other nurses and healthcare professionals to promote improved healthcare outcomes for patients and families in a variety of settings. Nursing accrediting bodies and professional nursing organizations have advocated for nurse practitioners to obtain a clinical doctoral degree in nursing, the DNP.

References

American Association of Colleges of Nursing. (2006). *The essentials of doctoral education for advanced nursing practice.* Retrieved from https://www.aacnnursing.org/Portals/42/Publications/DNPEssentials.pdf

American Association of Colleges of Nursing. (2011). *The essentials of master's education in nursing.* Retrieved from http://www.aacnnursing.org/portals/42/publications/mastersessentials11.pdf

American Association of Nurse Practitioners. (n.d.). *State practice environment.* Retrieved from https://www.aanp.org/advocacy/state/state-practice-environment

Association of American Medical Colleges. (2019). *New findings confirm predictions on physician shortage.* Retrieved from https://www.aamc.org/news-insights/press-releases/new-findings-confirm-predictions-physician-shortage

Ford, L. (1979). *Changing patterns in healthcare and the nurses' emerging role.* Bundoora, VIC, Australia: Preston Institute of Technology.

McCleery, E., Christensen, V., Peterson, K., Humphrey, L., & Helfand, M. (2014). *Evidence brief: The quality of care provided by advanced practice nurses.* Retrieved from https://www.ncbi.nlm.nih.gov/books/NBK 384613/

National Organization of Nurse Practitioner Faculties. (2018). *The doctor of nursing practice degree: Entry to nurse practitioner practice by 2025.* Retrieved from https://cdn.ymaws.com/www.nonpf.org/resource/ resmgr/dnp/v3_05.2018_NONPF_DNP_Stateme.pdf

Schveitzer, M., Zoboli, E., & Vieira, M. (2016). Nursing challenges for universal health coverage: A systematic review. *Revista Latino-Americana de Enfermagem, 24,* e2676. doi:10.1590/1518-8345.0933.2676

U.S. Centers for Medicare & Medicaid Services. (n.d.). *National health expenditure data: Historical.* Retrieved from https://www.cms.gov/ Research-Statistics-Data-and-Systems/Statistics-Trends-and-Reports/ NationalHealthExpendData/NationalHealthAccountsHistorical

2

The Intersection of Nursing, Medicine, and Public Health

Nursing has been referred to as both an art and a science. In order to maintain competency in providing high-quality healthcare to patients and families across the life span, healthcare providers must remain active in clinical practice. It is typical for healthcare professionals to keep abreast of these changes via reading, conferences, and webinars. However, evidence suggests that direct, hands-on clinical practice is the most effective way to gather knowledge in the health sciences (Giddens et al., 2014). Healthcare professionals must be recognized for their ability to solve global, complex healthcare challenges in interdisciplinary, collaborative ways. Nurses are uniquely poised to provide solutions to challenging problems. We communicate and work alongside all members of the multidisciplinary healthcare team in a meaningful and effective manner.

INTERDISCIPLINARY PRACTICE

Nurses with graduate degrees are at the forefront of preparing the future workforce of nurses and APRNs, both at the bedside and out in community-based settings. Newer nurses, in increasing numbers, are being encouraged to pursue advanced nursing degrees sooner than ever before to help meet the needs of today's ever-changing, ever-challenged healthcare system (Aktan, 2010, 2015). Related disciplines, such as areas in medicine and public health, partner with nursing professionals in the provision of timely, quality, and cost-effective healthcare outcomes by the collaborative promotion of health at the local, regional, national, and international levels.

The Value of Nursing as a Member of the Interdisciplinary Team

Nursing professionals serve as the primary contact with and advocate for patients, families, and communities. They play a key role in responding to the needs of individuals and populations and identifying issues affecting the health and well-being of their patients.

Fast Facts

Nurses and APRNs are responsible for discerning patterns across patient populations, linking patients with community resources and social services, and developing broad-based nursing and advanced practice nursing interventions (American Association of Colleges of Nursing [AACN], 2016; Bachrach & Thomas, 2016).

There is a need for nursing, public health, medical, business, government, and educational institutions to collaborate to train the current and future workforce to develop and apply evidence into effective interventions and monitor these outcomes. It has been well documented that research helps healthcare providers improve the practice. Efforts are needed to collect and disseminate information on the most effective evidence-based interventions. Nurse scientists bring a unique combination of clinical insight and practical experience integral to sustaining and advancing health, are skillful in basic scientific discovery, and are able to translate this knowledge into healthcare initiatives. The educational advancement of nurses, and all members of the multidisciplinary healthcare team, is essential to promote enhanced healthcare outcomes (Bachrach, Robert, & Thomas, 2015).

POPULATION HEALTH

Our nation's healthcare crisis requires broad changes. One such way our system is evolving is the examination and management of health at the population level. Population health, or addressing the health outcomes of a group of individuals, focuses on the assessment of health and health outcomes of whole groups of people and the unequal distribution of health across various subgroups (Kindig & Stoddart, 2003). The Institute of Medicine (IOM; now the National Academy of Medicine) has described population health as an approach that treats the population as a whole as the patient, which involves applying health strategies, interventions, and policies at the population level rather than through the episodic, individual-level actions common within acute care (IOM, 2014).

Fast Facts

The management of population health involves a range of activities such as the promotion of health and wellness and the prevention of disease. Goals include keeping the patient population as healthy as possible, minimizing the need for acute care interventions such as emergency department visits and hospitalizations, and reducing total cost. Collaborative areas to target include the following:

- higher levels of physical activity;
- declines in newly diagnosed cases of diabetes;
- lower preterm births and infant mortality; and
- fewer work days lost to illness/disability (Bolton & Anderson, 2014; IOM, 2014; Kindig, 2007; Watson Dillon, & Mahoney, 2015).

To adopt a public health management approach, organizations must adjust the organizational mission, take advantage of changes in reimbursement mechanisms, address changes in healthcare, and meet the expectations of community partners (McGuire, 2016). Future recommendations to improve population health incorporate the interfacing between system, individual, family, and community; identifying issues affecting health and well-being and patterns across patient populations; helping link community resources and social services and develop broad-based interventions; having opportunities to train nurses to function and thrive in transformed healthcare systems; addressing population health for students and retraining nurses currently in the workforce; focusing a shift away from the illness-focused acute care skills; expanding nursing fundamentals in health assessment, pathophysiology, and patient care; developing material focused on assisting the individual/family to achieve the highest level of functioning; and communicating with individuals, families, and the community (AACN, 2013; Bachrach & Thomas, 2016; Fraher, Spetz, & Naylor, 2015).

Nursing Program Gaps

Nursing professionals need greater educational preparation in the following areas: population health competencies, coordinating with interprofessional teams, understanding care as value-based with a focus across the life span, using ambulatory care delivery models, recognizing and responding to epidemiologic patterns, and study/analysis of the distribution, patterns, and determinants of health and disease conditions in populations (Calhoun & Harris, 2016). Keys to success involve competency in the support of complex patient groups, provision of care coordination, analysis of population-level data from electronic health records and other sources, and optimization of the use of research to promote evidence-based care. As many nurses and APRNs rate themselves as unprepared to conduct population-level assessment, evaluation, and research, policies and programs to better prepare nursing students in population health must include the following: population health concepts in curricula, testing, and licensure, training nurses in practice through continuing education, and providing certification in population health competencies (AACN, 2013; Fraher et al., 2015; Issel & Bekemeier, 2010).

Furthermore, there is a need for interdisciplinary accreditation standards. Courses from disciplines such as public health or social work must be included in nursing and advanced practice nursing education to help students understand the biological, social, political, economic, and environmental underpinnings of health and introduce the scientific framework of population health. Content must be expanded to focus on health equity, more sophisticated community health assessment, advanced epidemiologic methods, and ways to bridge clinical care and population health (Bachrach & Thomas, 2016).

Evolving Healthcare Roles

The jobs of nurses and other healthcare providers are changing dramatically. Healthcare professionals are assuming expanded roles in ambulatory care and community-based settings. Responsibilities are in population health, care coordination, and interprofessional collaboration. These have the potential to influence population health at all levels, including individual and institutional care and healthcare policy. Population health must include moving the healthcare system toward community-based preventive and proactive approaches. Nursing professionals need to take on roles as care coordinators, case managers, and transition specialists working with and leading teams that include physicians, pharmacists, social workers, and dieticians. Examples include coordinators, informatics specialists, community-based facilitators, and primary care partners (Fraher et al., 2015).

Rural and Underserved Areas

Nurses and APRNs may be the only health professionals serving clients in some rural and underserved areas. Attracting and retaining health professionals in remote areas presents many challenges. Rural residents tend to have higher rates of poverty and chronic disease, lower levels of health insurance coverage, riskier health behaviors, and more difficult access to healthcare than residents in urban areas (Buck, Crawford, Gale, Holzmark, & Mills, 2015). All members of the interdisciplinary healthcare team must assume a role in the identification of healthcare needs in at-risk populations and promote the meeting of such needs in order to reduce, or possibly diminish, these health disparities.

Technology

Technology plays a key role in the promotion of population health. Telecommunication technology can be used to advance health, and telehealth helps nurses and other healthcare professionals monitor health status, provide consultation, and offer health education. Texting-based services or mobile apps have been shown to contribute to improved healthcare outcomes. Examples include using text messages to promote prenatal care and to remind patients with congestive heart failure to take their medications. Some barriers limiting the use of telehealth are presented in Box 2.1.

Leadership

Nurse leaders must remain active and innovative in addressing the unique healthcare needs of a range of different populations. Evidence-based, nurse-led programs have led to improved healthcare outcomes. Nurses have been known to transform the healthcare industry, serve as champion advocates for improving community

BOX 2.1 TELEHEALTH BARRIERS

- A lack of reimbursement to providers
- Licensure requirements across state or other boundaries
- Workforce preparation and training
- Cost-effectiveness
- Expansion of the use of telehealth requires improving the skills of the workforce

Source: Data from Advisory Committee on Interdisciplinary, Community-Based Linkages. (2013). *Redesigning health professions education and practice to prepare the interprofessional team to care for populations* (12th Report). Rockville, MD: Health Resources and Services Administration; Bergeron, quoted in Lynch, J. P. (2016). Transforming primary care: One nurse's story. *Nurse.com, 1*(3), 24; Institute of Medicine. (2014). *Population health implications of the Affordable Care Act: Workshop summary*. Washington, DC: National Academies Press.

health, and build networks of resources and relationships due to skills in assessing the community needs, planning and implementing strategies, fostering trust, and managing changes in healthcare delivery. Nursing leadership must be cultivated to promote the necessary changes in nursing education and nursing practice, continue to foster a holistic nursing approach, develop robust data management skills, obtain funding to promote positive healthcare outcomes, and gather support of policy makers. The evidence suggests that these efforts will produce high-quality healthcare outcomes contributing to the reverse of the decline in health status and a decrease in the escalating costs of healthcare.

Fast Facts

- Newer nurses, in increasing numbers, are being encouraged to pursue advanced nursing degrees sooner than ever before to help meet the needs of today's ever-changing, ever-challenged healthcare system
- There is a need for nursing, public health, medical, business, government, and educational institutions to collaborate to train the current and future workforce to develop and apply the evidence into effective interventions and monitor these outcomes.
- Population health, or addressing the health outcomes of a group of individuals, focuses on the assessment of health and health outcomes of whole groups of people and the unequal distribution of health across various subgroups.
- Interdisciplinary accreditation standards must be developed to include expanded content focusing on health equity, more sophisticated community health assessment, advanced epidemiologic methods, and ways to bridge clinical care and population health.
- The jobs of nurses and other healthcare providers are changing dramatically, and healthcare professionals are assuming expanded roles in ambulatory care and community-based settings.
- All members of the interdisciplinary healthcare team must assume a role in the identification of healthcare needs in at-risk populations and promote the meeting of such needs in order to reduce, or possibly diminish, these health disparities.
- Technology plays a key role in the promotion of population health.
- Evidence-based, nurse-led programs have led to improved healthcare outcomes.

SUMMARY

As nursing professionals, we must commit to lifelong learning, be visionary, identify the necessary tools, data, and resources to improve care, and develop and implement critical communication and leadership skills. With over 244,000 APRNs in the United States today, and 80% of them practicing in primary care, all APRNs and our colleagues in related disciplines must contribute effectively to the provision of high-quality primary care services and function at the top of our license, as healthcare resources are scarce.

References

American Association of Colleges of Nursing. (2013). *Public health: Recommended baccalaureate competencies and curricular guidelines for public health nursing.* Washington, DC: Author.

American Association of Colleges of Nursing. (2016). *Advancing healthcare transformation: A new era for academic nursing.* Washington, DC: Author.

Aktan, N. (2010). *Fast facts for the new nurse practitioner: What you really need to know in a nutshell.* New York, NY: Springer Publishing Company.

Aktan, N. (2015). *Fast facts for the new nurse practitioner: What you really need to know in a nutshell* (2nd ed.). New York, NY: Springer Publishing Company.

Bachrach, C., Robert, S., & Thomas, Y. (2015). *Training in interdisciplinary health science: Current successes and future needs.* Institute of Medicine Roundtable on Population Health Improvement. Washington, DC: National Academies Press.

Bachrach, C., & Thomas, Y. (2016, June). *Training nurses in population health science: What, why, how?* Presentation at the 133rd meeting of the National Advisory Council for Nurse Education and Practice, Rockville, MD.

Bolton, L. B., & Anderson, R. (2014). Population health management. *Nursing Administration Quarterly, 38*(2), 105–106. doi:10.1097/NAQ.0000000000 000028

Buck, S., Crawford, P. A., Gale, J., Holzmark, D., & Milles, M. (2015). *National Rural Health Association policy brief: Population health in rural communities.* Washington, DC: National Rural Health Association.

Calhoun, B., & Harris, K. (2016, January). *The promise of nursing in population health: The experience of Banner Health.* Presentation at the 133rd meeting of the National Advisory Council for Nurse Education and Practice, Rockville, MD.

Fraher, E., Spetz, J., & Naylor, M. (2015). *Nursing in a transformed health care system: New roles, new rules.* Robert Wood Johnson Foundation Interdisciplinary Nursing Quality Research Initiative. Retrieved from http://ldi.upenn.edu/brief/nursing-transformed-health-care-system-new -roles-new-rules

Giddens, J., Lauson-Clabo, L., Morton, P., Jeffries, P., McQuade-Jones, B., & Ryan, S. (2014). Re-envisioning clinical education for nurse practitioner programs: Themes from a national leaders' dialogue. *Journal of Professional Nursing, 30*(3), 273–278. doi:10.1016/j.profnurs.2014.03.002

Institute of Medicine. (2014). *Population health implications of the Affordable Care Act: Workshop summary.* Washington, DC: National Academies Press.

Issel, L. M., & Bekemeier, B. (2010). Safe practice of population-focused nursing care: Development of a public health nursing concept. *Nursing Outlook, 58,* 226–232. doi:10.1016/j.outlook.2010.06.001

Kindig, D., & Stoddart, G. (2003). What is population health? *American Journal of Public Health, 93,* 380–383. doi:10.2105/AJPH.93.3.380

Kindig, D. A. (2007). Understanding population health terminology. *The Milbank Quarterly, 85*(1), 139–161. doi:10.1111/j.1468-0009.2007.00479.x

McGuire, J. F.; Northeastern University Institute on Urban Health Research and Practice. (2016). *Population Health Investments by Health Plans and Large Provider Organizations – Exploring the Business Case.* Retrieved from the Northeastern University website: https://www.northeastern.edu/iuhrp/wp-content/uploads/2016/05/PopHealthBusinessCaseFullRpt-5-1.pdf

Watson Dillon, D. M., & Mahoney, M. A. (2015). Moving from patient care to population health: A new competency for the executive nurse leader. *Nurse Leader, 13*(1), 30–32, 36. doi:10.1016/j.mnl.2014.11.002

3

Practice Essentials for Allergy and Immunology

Clients often seek care for allergic symptoms in primary care settings. At times, this is appropriate, and symptoms are managed appropriately with optimal outcomes achieved. More severe or difficult-to-control conditions should be referred to a specialist or emergency services when indicated. Evidence suggests that allergies are underdiagnosed in primary care settings and that inappropriate management has been shown to significantly impact the quality of life (Demoly et al., 2019).

ALLERGY MANAGEMENT

Acute Allergic Reaction to Food

Clients often present to primary care settings reporting an actual or potential allergic reaction to a certain food(s). Most typically, food allergy symptoms are rapid in onset after ingesting the food (within 2 hours and rarely within 8 hours) and can potentially be facilitated by physical exercise, ingestion of nonsteroidal anti-inflammatory drugs, alcohol, stress, or infection. Symptoms may not improve with time from food intake (Demoly et al., 2019).

When the presenting client has no evidence of anaphylaxis or is symptomatic in one organ system only with one suspected trigger food, an emergency kit without epinephrine is to be prescribed (except in cases with associated asthma), education to avoid suspected food is provided, and specific immunoglobulin E (IgE) assays are conducted. If these tests are positive, the client is to be referred to a specialist; however, if these tests are negative, the client's symptoms are unlikely related to a food allergy. In the case of severe anaphylaxis or severe allergic symptoms affecting two or more organs, the client should be referred to emergency care when indicated, sent to an allergist for risk assessment and management, instructed on food avoidance, and prescribed an emergency kit with epinephrine and instructed on its use (Demoly et al., 2019).

Allergic Respiratory Symptoms

Clients also often present to primary care settings reporting allergic respiratory symptoms. When the respiratory symptoms are chronic in nature or recurring, there is evidence of exposure to allergic triggers, symptoms are impairing the quality of life and are not controlled by first-line treatments, and/or two or more systems are affected, it is appropriate to conduct blood screening test for a respiratory allergy. If such testing is negative, then the provider must search for other nonallergic causes of the symptoms. If the blood test is positive, the skillful provider must initiate or adapt the management plan or consult with a specialist. If symptoms persist or if polysensitization has occurred, then a referral to an allergist is indicated. Furthermore, it is imperative to implement environmental control measures if called for by the patient's medical history and specific IgE assays (Demoly et al., 2019).

Acute Allergic Reactions to Drugs

Clients also often present to primary care settings reporting an actual or potential acute allergic reaction to a pharmacologic agent. The appearance of symptoms, both on the treatment or when stopping treatment, is important for the provider to note. The presence of a rash (e.g., macules, papules, vesicles) with or without urticaria, combined with respiratory (e.g., rhinoconjunctivitis, nasal itching, runny nose, nasal obstruction, red itching eyes, watering eyes, asthma, dyspnea, chest tightness, wheezing), digestive (e.g., oropharyngeal itching, mouth edema, nausea, vomiting, abdominal pain, abdominal distention, abdominal noises, diarrhea), and cardiovascular (e.g., tachycardia, hypotension) symptoms, may indicate reaction severity (Demoly et al., 2019).

Fast Facts

It is critical to assess for the rapid disappearance of a rash after stopping medication. In any unknown chronology of the allergic response or in the case of a more severe reaction, a referral to an allergist is indicated.

The criteria in favor of an alternate diagnosis include the following: The medication is taken since the initial reaction without a subsequent reaction, and the symptoms appear without taking the drug. A picture should be taken and documented if an allergic reaction is expected (Demoly et al., 2019).

Immunotherapy

Immunotherapy is the practice of exposing patients to a specific allergen in order to promote tolerance to that allergen and control a sustained decrease in the reaction (Aiken, 2014). This practice aims to sustain the immune response after the discontinuation of the treatment. Subcutaneous immunotherapy is the most popular allergy treatment method in the United States today (Aiken, 2014).

Currently, allergen immunotherapy consists of two phases of buildup and maintenance. Buildup involves increasing one to two weekly doses of the extract until a therapeutically effective maintenance dosage is reached. Then, after the maintenance dosage is reached, the interval between dosages is gradually increased. It has been reported that maintenance therapy continues for 3 to 5 years in duration for the best long-term benefits. As a great number of allergic patients are seen in primary care settings, and there is a projected decrease in allergists, the majority of allergic conditions may be treated in primary care settings (Aiken, 2014).

ASTHMA

It has been reported that the number of clients with allergic diseases such as asthma continues to grow. In 2001, 20 million patients had asthma in the United States, compared with 25 million in 2009 (or 8% of the population; Demoly et al., 2019). Education is the hallmark of improved outcomes in the management of the asthmatic client, and strategies for better asthmatic control are summarized by Demoly et al. (2019) and are provided in Box 3.1.

The skillful primary care provider is savvy to incorporate these critical elements of asthma education into the comprehensive management plan (Boulet et al., 2015). The difficult-to-manage asthmatic client should consult with a specialty provider. Examples include an allergist and/or a pulmonologist.

The evidence suggests that a referral to a specialty provider may promote improved outcomes in the asthmatic client. An allergist/immunologist will evaluate for the need to perform challenge testing for confirmation of airway reactivity, the role of allergy (IgE history), and/or occupational exposures to decrease emergency department

BOX 3.1 STRATEGIES TO CONTROL ASTHMA

- Smoking cessation
- Environmental control
- Use of an action plan
- Knowledge and understanding of the disease, including pathophysiology
- Pathophysiology
- Symptoms of an exacerbation
- Importance of medication adherence
- Inhaler technique and proper use of spirometry

visits/hospitalizations and minimize potential for fatal asthma outcomes, particularly in those with prior severe life-threatening episodes. To improve outcomes, clients with moderate-to-severe persistent asthma, clients with symptoms of uncontrolled asthma in spite of therapy, clients who use excessive amounts of rescue medications (1 canister per month or more), clients with suboptimal adherence or self-management, or clients with associated rhinitis or sinusitis should also be referred to an allergist/immunologist (American Academy of Allergy, Asthma & Immunology, n.d.).

ALLERGIC RHINITIS

Clients commonly present to primary care settings reporting rhinitis. Anticipated triggers include indoor and outdoor allergens such as dust mites, insects, animal dander, molds, and pollen, and symptoms include rhinorrhea, sneezing, nasal congestion, nasal obstruction, and nasal pruritus. Current evidence suggests that the initial treatment should include intranasal corticosteroids alone when symptoms affect quality of life; more severe cases that do not respond to intranasal corticosteroids should be treated with second-generation antihistamines that cause less sedation and have a lower adverse event profile (with the exception of cetirizine) or oral leukotriene receptor antagonists (particularly effective in clients with coexistent asthma); and in cases of moderate-to-severe persistent symptoms that are unresponsive to treatment, the skillful primary care practitioner should consider referral for immunotherapy. Studies do not support the use of nasal decongestants for more than 3 days due to rebound congestion, mite-proof mattresses/pillow covers, breastfeeding, air filtration systems, or delayed exposure to solid foods in infancy or to pets in childhood to treat or reduce allergic symptoms (Sur & Plesa, 2015).

URTICARIA

Clients also commonly present to primary care settings complaining of urticaria. Various etiologies may include infection (e.g., sinusitis, tonsillitis, dental abscess, urinary tract infection, hepatitis, infectious mononucleosis, parasites), medicines (e.g., see the Fast Facts box in this section summarizing these), food (e.g., nuts, eggs, seafood, fish, chocolate, meat, cow's milk, fruits, vegetables, fermented foods, spices, spirits), psychogenic factors (e.g., stress, sadness, depression), physical factors (e.g., pressure, hot, cold), or respiratory allergens (e.g., pollen, mold spores, mites, animal dandruff, hair). At times, the cause may be idiopathic or hereditary. Systemic diseases, such as thyroid, or rheumatologic diseases, such as systemic lupus erythematosus, lymphoma, leukemia, and carcinomas, may present with chronic urticaria, and latex, cosmetics, and chemicals may cause contact urticaria (Kayiran & Akdeniz, 2019).

Fast Facts

The following medications may result in urticaria:

- Penicillin
- Sulfonamides
- Angiotensin-converting enzyme inhibitors
- Morphine
- Aspirin
- Thiazide diuretics
- Vitamins
- Nonsteroidal anti-inflammatory drugs
- Oral contraceptives
- Codeine

Although the client most often describes pruritic, red, swollen, itchy plaques that often resolve spontaneously within 2 to 3 hours, at times the episode may involve angioedema, including swelling of the lips and eyelids, which can affect the respiratory tract. When the respiratory tract is involved, the episode may be life-threatening and care is urgent. The preferred treatment is antihistamines and systemic corticosteroids; however, H2 antagonists may be added for resistant symptoms. The elimination of the etiologic agent and avoidance of triggers play an integral role in management (Kayiran & Akdeniz, 2019).

- In the case of severe anaphylaxis or severe allergic symptoms affecting two or more organs, the client should be referred to emergency care when indicated, sent to an allergist for risk assessment and management, instructed on food avoidance, and prescribed an emergency kit with epinephrine and instructed on its use.

- When the allergic respiratory symptoms are chronic in nature or recurring, there is evidence of exposure to allergic triggers, symptoms are impairing the quality of life and are not controlled by first-line treatments, and/or two or more systems are affected, it is appropriate to conduct blood screening test for a respiratory allergy.

- The criteria in favor of an alternate diagnosis beyond an allergic reaction to a medication include the following: The medication is taken since the initial reaction without a subsequent reaction, and the symptoms appear without taking the drug.

- Immunotherapy is the practice of exposing patients to a specific allergen in order to promote tolerance to that allergen and control a sustained decrease in the reaction.

- To improve outcomes, clients with moderate-to-severe persistent asthma, clients with symptoms of uncontrolled asthma in spite of therapy, clients who use excessive amounts of rescue medications (1 canister per month or more), clients with suboptimal adherence or self-management, or clients with associated rhinitis or sinusitis should also be referred to an allergist/immunologist.

- Current evidence suggests that the initial treatment for allergic rhinitis should include intranasal corticosteroids alone when symptoms affect the quality of life; more severe cases that do not respond to intranasal corticosteroids should be treated with second-generation antihistamines that cause less sedation and have a lower adverse event profile (with the exception of cetirizine) or oral leukotriene receptor antagonist (particularly effective in clients with coexistent asthma); and in cases of moderate-to-severe persistent symptoms that are unresponsive to treatment, the skillful primary care practitioner should consider referral for immunotherapy.

- The preferred treatment for urticaria is antihistamines and systemic corticosteroids; however, H2 antagonists may be added for resistant symptoms.

SUMMARY

This journey through the subspecialties continued with a variety of collaborative clinical practice sessions with physician specialists and nurse practitioners practicing in specialty settings. Clients presented with common allergic/immunologic complaints that often begin with their visit to the primary care provider. This clinical immersion experience led to the identification of hot topics that the primary/urgent care nurse practitioner is expected to diagnose or perhaps initiate management of. As always, effective management plans can only be developed once the provider has identified the correct etiology.

References

Aiken, B. (2014). Majority of allergies can be treated in primary care. *Clinical Advisor.* Retrieved from https://www.clinicaladvisor.com/home/meeting-coverage/aanp-2014/majority-of-allergies-can-be-treated-in-primary-care/

American Academy of Allergy, Asthma & Immunology. (n.d.). *Primary care summary.* Retrieved from https://www.aaaai.org/practice-resources/consultation-and-referral-guidelines/primary-care-summary

Boulet, L., Boulay, M., Gauthier, G., Battisti, L., Chabot, V., Beauchesne, M., & Cote, P. (2015). Benefits of an asthma education program provided at primary care sites on asthma outcomes. *Respiratory Medicine, 109*, 991–1000. doi:10.1016/j.rmed.2015.05.004

Demoly, P., Chabane, H., Fontaine, J., Boissieu, D., Ryan, D., Angier, E., & Just, J. (2019). Development of algorithms for the diagnosis and management of acute allergy in primary practice. *The World Allergy Organization Journal, 12*(3), 100022. doi:10.1016/j.waojou.2019.100022

Kayiran, M., & Akdeniz, N. (2019). Diagnosis and treatment of urticaria in primary care. *Northern Clinics of Istanbul, 6*(1), 93–99. doi:10.14744/nci.2018.75010

Sur, D., & Plesa, M. (2015). Treatment of allergic rhinitis. *American Family Physician, 92*(11), 985–992.

4

Practice Essentials for Cardiology

This journey through the subspecialties continues with some of the most common complaints that result in the client's visit to the primary care provider—disorders of the cardiovascular system. Although many of these conditions require consultation with a cardiologist and/or other specialty provider, it is often the primary care provider who is first faced with the diagnosis and management of common cardiac conditions. As always, effective management plans can only be developed once the provider has identified the correct condition.

PREVENTION OF CARDIAC DISEASE IN PRIMARY CARE

The mainstay of primary care efforts must be directed toward the prevention of morbidity and mortality related to cardiac conditions. This is an essential role of the primary care provider. A number of chronic conditions can be managed, or perhaps eliminated, when clients comply with key lifestyle modifications.

Obesity in America

Nationwide, 39.6% of adults were considered obese in 2015 to 2016, the highest percentages ever documented. Primary care providers play a key role in the management of obesity. It is important to identify this health concern and discuss the implications with the patient. Seasoned practitioners know what types of resources are available in the community so that they can refer patients as needed and are prepared to discuss changes in diet that patients are likely to try and willing to adopt (State of Childhood Obesity, n.d.).

Furthermore, proper diabetic, hypertension, and hyperlipidemia management are critical elements of overall cardiovascular health. The Dietary Approaches to Stop Hypertension (DASH) diet is a flexible, balanced plan that helps create a heart-healthy eating style for life (National Heart, Lung, and Blood Institute, n.d.). This plan requires no special foods. The DASH diet provides daily and weekly nutritional goals, and recommendations are provided in Box 4.1:

BOX 4.1   DIETARY APPROACHES TO STOP HYPERTENSION DIET RECOMMENDATIONS

Vegetables	Fruits	Whole grains
Fat-free or low-fat dairy products	Fish	Poultry
Beans	Nuts	Vegetable oils
Limited foods that are high in saturated fat, such as fatty meats	Limited full-fat dairy products	Limited tropical oils, such as coconut, palm kernel, and palm oils
Limited sugar-sweetened beverages	Limited sweets	

The DASH eating plan targets for a 2,000-calorie-a-day diet while choosing foods that are low in saturated and trans fats, rich in potassium, calcium, magnesium, fiber, and protein, and lower in sodium. Studies showed that the DASH diet may lower blood pressure and low-density lipoprotein cholesterol (LDL-C) significantly (National Heart, Lung, and Blood Institute, n.d.).

Importance of Physical Activity

The primary care provider should gather data on activity levels and provide education on the current guidelines for physical activity to the adult client. The adult client should be instructed to move more and sit less throughout the day.

Fast Facts

For substantial health benefits, adults should be educated to do at least 150 to 300 minutes a week of moderate-intensity or 75 to 150 minutes a week of vigorous-intensity aerobic physical activity.

(continued)

(continued)

For additional health benefits, the practitioner should also promote that the adult client does muscle-strengthening activities of moderate or greater intensity that involve all major muscle groups on two or more days a week (U.S. Department of Health and Human Services, n.d.).

Nicotine Product Cessation

The primary care provider should also gather data on the use of nicotine products and provide education on the current guidelines for cessation to the adult client. The recommended algorithm to address smoking habits with clients who are current smokers includes the following four tasks: (a) assessment, (b) advice to quit, (c) offer and provide treatment, and (d) follow up (http://www.onlinejacc .org/content/72/25/33320). The Federal Drug Administration has approved nicotine replacement therapy (NRT), bupropion, and varenicline for smoking cessation. All are tolerable and effective options for healthy smokers, as well as for those clients with stable cardiovascular disease. Studies indicate that varenicline and combination NRT are more effective than bupropion or single NRT products alone, making these two approaches first-line recommendations for smoking cessation. Single NRT and bupropion should be considered second-line therapies. Combinations of agents may be recommended for smokers who have only a partial response or who fail to achieve complete tobacco abstinence with individual agents alone (https://www.onlinejacc.org/content/74/10/e177).

Limitation of Alcoholic Intake

The primary care practitioner should also gather data on alcoholic intake and provide education on the current guidelines for the adult client as they relate to cardiovascular health. There are a number of acute and chronic health conditions related to the abuse of alcohol. For instance, studies reflect the lowest risk of myocardial infarction (MI) in adult clients who consume one alcoholic beverage per day or less. In addition, the research on heavy drinkers demonstrates dramatic increase in blood pressure—a risk factor for both MI and congestive heart failure (CHF). Furthermore, there is a known association between alcohol abuse and left ventricular dysfunction (Criqui & Thomas, 2017). Overall, alcohol is dangerous to the cardiovascular, as well as a number of other body systems, and patient counseling regarding risk and strategies for cessation is the mainstay of primary care practice. Alcohol should be consumed in moderation and only in accordance with the current guidelines—up to one alcoholic beverage per day for women and up to two for men (Centers for Disease Control and Prevention, n.d.).

Stress Management

The primary care provider should gather data on a client's stress levels and provide education on the importance of and strategies for stress reduction and stress management. Stress reduction is an important element of overall health. Principles of cardiovascular health incorporate lifestyle practices, where stress levels are perceived as manageable by the adult client.

It has been reported that psychological stress contributes to the long-term development of coronary heart disease and the acute triggering of cardiac events. Furthermore, chronic stress is associated with a 40% to 50% increase in the occurrence of coronary heart disease, and long-term stress is associated with poor prognosis among patients with established coronary heart disease (Steptoe & Kivimake, 2012). Studies have documented that workplace stress, financial stress, caregiver stress, or disaster-related stress can impact cardiac health, and strategies, such as the promotion of adequate sleep and regular exercise, and relaxation techniques, such as meditation, progressive muscle relaxation, guided imagery, deep breathing exercises, and yoga, can be used effectively to manage stress (Harvard Health Publishing, n.d.). The skillful primary care provider not only gathers data on a client's stress levels and current practices to manage stress but is also prepared to discuss evidence-based recommendations for stress reduction and offer resources to ensure the client is able to effectively cope with acute and chronic stressors.

MANAGEMENT OF CARDIAC DISEASE IN PRIMARY CARE

It is imperative to be clear that the primary care provider acknowledge that acute cardiac pathology is managed in emergency settings alone. There are, however, a number of common chronic cardiac conditions that are appropriately managed by the skillful provider in primary care settings. Examples include the management of the low-risk hypertensive client or the client with hyperlipidemia. Others involve controlled cardiac conditions such as certain arrhythmias or CHF. It is imperative that the practitioner is mindful of the limitations of managing uncontrolled cardiac disease in primary care settings and refer the client to a specialty provider when indicated and appropriate.

Hypertension

It is often the primary care provider who first encounters the client with undiagnosed hypertension. Initial diagnosis and management are integral roles of the primary care provider. For proper assessment of blood pressure, the client should be relaxed and sitting in a chair with feet on the floor, having avoided caffeine, exercise, or smoking for at least 30 minutes prior to measurement.

Fast Facts

Elevated blood pressure is characterized as systolic blood pressure (SBP) 120 to 129 mm Hg and diastolic blood pressure (DBP) >80 mm Hg; stage 1 hypertension is categorized as SBP 130 to 139 or DBP 80 to 89, and stage 2 hypertension is diagnosed with the blood pressure ≥140/90 (Whelton & Carey, 2018).

The seasoned provider considers the cause of the hypertension (e.g., genetic, environmental, obesity, sodium intake, level of physical fitness, or alcohol intake) prior to the initiation of the appropriate therapy. Furthermore, it is critical to consider causes of secondary hypertension such as renal disease, primary aldosteronism, obstructive sleep apnea, or drug-/alcohol-induced conditions (e.g., amphetamines, antidepressants, caffeine, decongestants, oral contraceptives, nonsteroidal anti-inflammatory drugs, corticosteroids, herbal supplements, systemic corticosteroids, or immunosuppressant agents). Although relatively uncommon, other causes may include Cushing's syndrome, thyroid disorders, or primary hyperparathyroidism (Whelton & Carey, 2018).

Laboratory measurements should be obtained for clients newly diagnosed with hypertension to determine risk, establish a baseline for medication management, and screen for secondary causes of hypertension. Initial basic testing includes blood glucose, complete blood count, lipid profile, serum creatinine, sodium, potassium, and calcium levels, thyroid-stimulating hormone, urinalysis, and electrocardiogram. Optional testing may include echocardiogram, uric acid level, and urinary albumin-to-creatinine ratio (Whelton & Carey, 2018).

BOX 4.2 NONPHARMACOLOGICAL HYPERTENSION MANAGEMENT

- Weight management
- Sodium restriction
- Increased physical activity
- Initiation of a heart-healthy diet
- Potassium supplementation unless contraindicated
- Minimization of alcohol intake

Source: Data from Whelton, P., & Carey, R. (2018). 2017 ACC/AHA/AAPA/ ABC/ACPM/AGS/APhA/ASH/ASPC/NMA/PCNA guideline for the prevention, detection, evaluation, and management of high blood pressure in adults. *Journal of the America College of Cardiology, 71*(19), e127–e248. doi:10.1016/j.jacc.2017.11.006

The management of the hypertensive client is the priority of the primary care clinician. Nonpharmacological interventions may be effective in lowering blood pressure. Key principles of the nonpharmacologic management of hypertension are summarized in Box 4.2 (Whelton & Carey, 2018).

Often, the pharmacologic management of hypertension is indicated. Antihypertensive agents are indicated for the client with blood pressure ≥140/90 and no history of cardiovascular disease or ≥130/80 for the client with clinical cardiovascular disease. The clinician must consider overall patient health with an emphasis on the reduction of future adverse cardiovascular outcomes while determining the pharmacologic management of hypertensive clients. A blood pressure target of <130/80 is recommended (Whelton & Carey, 2018).

First-line antihypertensive agents include thiazide diuretics, calcium channel blockers (CCBs), angiotensin-converting enzyme (ACE) inhibitors, or angiotensin II receptive blockers (ARBs), and monthly reevaluation should be conducted until blood pressure control is achieved. Five classes of antihypertensive agents have been shown to prevent cardiovascular disease: diuretics, ACE inhibitors, ARBs, CCBs, and β-blockers. Thiazide diuretics have been found to be superior in preventing heart failure over CCBs and ACE inhibitors. Additionally, ACE inhibitors were determined to be less effective than thiazide diuretics and CCBs in lowering blood pressure and in the prevention of stroke. In the general population, β-blockers were less effective than CCBs and thiazide diuretics in the reduction of stroke risk. Studies have also demonstrated that CCBs are as effective as diuretics in the reduction of cardiovascular events and are good initial choices when diuretic agents are not tolerated. Finally, an ARB may be better tolerated than ACE inhibitors in black patients, with less cough and angioedema, yet, evidence suggests that thiazide diuretics and CCBs are the best initial choice for single-drug therapy in this population. The majority of hypertensive clients are treated with more than one antihypertensive agent to achieve blood pressure control (Whelton & Carey, 2018).

Out-of-office blood pressure assessment and reporting plays a role in the determination of agent efficacy, minimizes the risk of white coat effect, and contributes positively to the achievement of blood pressure targets. The skillful practitioner incorporates education on the proper process for client self-monitoring and is conscientious to assess for the presence of adverse effects often experienced by clients who undergo antihypertensive therapy. These may interfere with medication adherence. Adverse effects include frequent micturition and headaches (CCBs); excessive micturition and dizziness (diuretics); dry irritating cough (ACE); and frequency of micturition, reduction in libido, and headaches (all) resulting in the discontinuation or substitution of therapy in 49.5% of patients (Olowofela & Isah, 2017). With proper assessment, thoughtful patient education, frequent evaluation, and substitution when indicated, unnecessary side effects can be minimized and compliance can be promoted.

Hyperlipidemia

Clients commonly present to primary care settings for the diagnosis and management of hyperlipidemia. Ideally, a healthy lifestyle reduces atherosclerotic cardiovascular disease (ASCVD) risk at all ages. In the younger adult client (aged 20–39 years), a healthy lifestyle promotes risk reduction, and assessment of lifetime risk facilitates the discussion of patient risk. For the adult client aged 40 to 75 years with diabetes mellitus, guidelines include the initiation of statin therapy with LDL-C >70 mg/dL, and for those without diabetes mellitus, discussion should include a review of major risk factors such as smoking, presence of hypertension, and the severity of the hyperlipidemia.

Fast Facts

In severe hyperlipidemia (LDC-C >190 mg/dL), the skilled provider is certain to initiate statin therapy regardless of the presence of additional risk factors and may consider adding ezetimibe as a secondary pharmacological agent (Grundy & Stone, 2019).

A coronary artery calcium (CAC) score, also called a coronary calcium scan, is a test that measures the amount of calcium in the walls of the heart's arteries. These deposits of calcium in the coronary arteries are a sign that there may also be a buildup of plaque making a heart attack or stroke more likely. This scan is one way to estimate someone's risk of developing heart disease or having a heart attack or stroke (American College of Cardiology, n.d.). If the CAC score is 0, treatment with statin therapy may be withheld or delayed, except in clients who smoke, present with comorbid diabetes mellitus, or have a strong family history of ASCVD. A score of 1 to 99 favors statin therapy, particularly in the client aged ≥55 years. In any client with a CAC >100, statin therapy is indicated (Grundy & Stone, 2019).

The seasoned practitioner conducts a focused assessment on overall cardiac risk. Other factors to consider in the decision-making to initiate statin therapy include a family history of premature ASCVD, persistently elevated LDL-C >160 mg/dL, presence of metabolic syndrome, chronic kidney disease, history of preeclampsia or premature menopause, chronic inflammatory disorders such as rheumatoid arthritis, high-risk ethnic groups (South Asian), or those with persistent elevations of triglycerides >175 mg/dL. It is critical to assess adherence and response to statin therapy and lifestyle changes with repeat lipid measurement 4 to 12 weeks after statin initiation or any dose adjustment and to repeat lipid measurement during 3 to 12 months' intervals and as needed (Grundy & Stone, 2019).

Heart Failure

The primary care clinician plays a key role in the recognition and investigation, referral to cardiologist for diagnosis, and management of the client in heart failure. Heart failure is a clinical syndrome characterized by certain signs and symptoms, plus objective evidence of a structural or functional abnormality of the heart. Often, the client presents with dyspnea, edema, orthopnea, and fatigue. The client history typically includes cardiovascular disease, particularly previous MI. On physical examination, signs may include crackles at the lung bases, a raised jugular venous pressure, or a displaced apex beat (Taylor, Rutten, Brouwer, & Hobbs, 2017).

As in all chronic conditions, a patient-centered approach to management is critical. Although at times hospitalization and/or care by a cardiologist or other specialist are required, clients with heart failure should understand their condition and be actively involved in management decisions, including aspects of self-care, as lifestyle interventions can improve patients' quality of life and prevent exacerbations. For instance, patients should be made aware of the role of salt and encouraged to avoid overuse, the importance of ensuring adequate hydration and a healthy diet, and the benefits of regular exercise in increasing their functional capacity (Taylor et al., 2017).

Medical management will likely include diuretics, as well as other pharmacologic agents. Diuretic therapy is critical in the initial phase of treatment to off-load fluid and improve symptoms. In addition, digoxin may be of use in patients with heart failure and atrial fibrillation to control ventricular rate. A new class of drug has recently been introduced to heart failure management options. Angiotensin receptor neprilysin inhibitors exert a dual action through inhibition of the renin–angiotensin system and potentiation of protective vasoactive neuropeptides. This class should be initiated only by a specialist. Primary care providers and specialists must work together to collaborate in providing patient-centered care, which optimizes both the quantity and quality of life in heart failure clients (Taylor et al., 2017).

Fast Facts

- Studies showed that the DASH diet may lower blood pressure and LDL-C significantly.
- For substantial health benefits, adults should be educated to do at least 150 to 300 minutes a week of moderate-intensity or 75 to 150 minutes a week of vigorous-intensity aerobic physical activity.
- Studies indicate that varenicline and combination NRT are more effective than bupropion or single NRT products alone, making these two approaches first-line recommendations for smoking cessation.
- Alcohol should be consumed in moderation and only in accordance with current guidelines—up to one alcoholic beverage per day for women and up to two for men.
- Psychological stress contributes to the long-term development of coronary heart disease and the acute triggering of cardiac events.
- First-line antihypertensive agents include thiazide diuretics, CCBs, ACE inhibitors, or ARBs, and monthly reevaluation should be conducted until blood pressure control is achieved.
- Factors to consider in decision-making to initiate statin therapy include family history of premature ASCVD, persistently elevated LDL-C >160 mg/dL, metabolic syndrome, chronic kidney disease, history of preeclampsia or premature menopause, chronic inflammatory disorders such as rheumatoid arthritis, high-risk ethnic groups, or those with persistent elevations of triglycerides >175 mg/dL.

SUMMARY

This journey through the subspecialties continued with a variety of collaborative clinical practice sessions with physician specialists and nurse practitioners practicing in specialty settings. Clients presented with common complaints that often begin with their visit to the primary care provider. This clinical immersion experience led to the identification of hot topics that the primary/urgent care nurse practitioner is expected to diagnose or perhaps initiate during the management of clients with cardiac conditions. As always, effective management plans can only be developed once the provider has identified the correct etiology.

References

American College of Cardiology. (n.d.). *Understanding coronary artery calcium (CAC) scoring*. Retrieved from https://www.cardiosmart.org/Heart-Conditions/High-Cholesterol/Content/Coronary-Artery-Calcium-Scoring

Centers for Disease Control and Prevention. (n.d.). *Frequently asked questions*. Retrieved from https://www.cdc.gov/alcohol/faqs.htm#okay

Criqui, M., & Thomas, I. (2017). Alcohol consumption and cardiac disease. *Journal of the American College of Cardiology, 69*(1), 25–27. doi:10.1016/j.jacc.2016.10.049

Grundy, S., & Stone, N. (2019). 2018 AHA/ACC/AACVPR/AAPA/ABC/ACPM/ADA/AGS/APhA/ASPC/NLA/PCNA guideline on the management of blood cholesterol. *Journal of the America College of Cardiology, 73*(24), e285-e350. doi:10.1016/j.jacc.2018.11.003

Harvard Health Publishing. (n.d.). *Reduce your stress to protect your heart*. Retrieved from https://www.health.harvard.edu/healthbeat/reduce-your-stress-to-protect-your-heart

National Heart, Lung, and Blood Institute. (n.d.). *DASH eating plan*. Retrieved from https://www.nhlbi.nih.gov/health-topics/dash-eating-plan

Olowofela, A., & Isah, A. (2017). A profile of adverse effects of antihypertensive medicines in a tertiary care clinic in Nigeria. *Annals of African Medicine, 16*(3), 114–119. doi:10.4103/aam.aam_6_17

State of Childhood Obesity. (n.d.). *Building a healthier future*. Retrieved from www.stateofobesity.org

Steptoe, A., & Kivimaki, M. (2012). Stress and cardiovascular disease. *Nature Reviews Cardiology, 9*, 360–370. doi:10.1038/nrcardio.2012.45

Taylor, C., Rutten, F., Brouwer, J., & Hobbs, R. (2017). Practical guidance on heart failure diagnosis and management in primary care: Recent EPCCS recommendations. *British Journal of General Practice, 67*(660), 326–327. doi:10.3399/bjgp17X691553

U.S. Department of Health and Human Services. (n.d.). *Physical activity guidelines for Americans: Executive summary.* Retrieved from https://health.gov/sites/default/files/2019-10/PAG_ExecutiveSummary.pdf

Whelton, P., & Carey, R. (2018). 2017 ACC/AHA/AAPA/ABC/ACPM/AGS/APhA/ASH/ASPC/NMA/PCNA guideline for the prevention, detection, evaluation, and management of high blood pressure in adults. *Journal of the America College of Cardiology, 71*(19), e127–e248. doi:10.1016/j.jacc.2017.11.006

5

Practice Essentials for Dermatology

The adult client may present to primary care settings with a variety of symptoms related to the dermatological system. Although many of these conditions are appropriate for the primary care provider to diagnose and manage, some conditions may be persistent or significant enough to be referred to the dermatologist. The skillful provider is knowledgeable on the standards of care for the client with a skin condition as well as the red flags to assess for and when to refer the patient for a consultation with a specialty provider.

ACNE VULGARIS

Clients may present to the primary care setting complaining of symptoms of acne. A thorough history includes discussion of symptoms that worsen related to the menstrual cycle, other triggers, endocrine abnormalities, and/or medication use that may be triggering symptoms such as corticosteroids, progestins, lithium, phenytoin, and iodides. In general, mild acne does not require systemic therapy. Moderate-to-severe symptoms likely require both topical (e.g., retinoids, antibiotics, keratolytics, or dapsone gel) and oral pharmacologic management (antibiotics such as erythromycin or tetracyclines, oral contraceptive, or isotretinoin). Here, a referral to a dermatologist may be indicated. Clients should be educated that it may take 6 to 12 weeks to note improvement (Consultant360, 2015). Table 5.1 presents grades I to IV of acne.

Table 5.1

Acne Grades	
Grade I	Mainly comedones
Grade II	Mixture of comedones and few inflammatory lesions
Grade III	Inflammatory papules and pustules
Grade IV	Nodulocystic, usually with scarring

ROSACEA

When the adult client presents to the primary care setting with recurrent episodes of facial flushing, erythema, papules, pustules, and telangiectasias, a diagnosis of rosacea should be considered. Although rosacea is a benign condition, symptoms can result in a decreased quality of life so that intervention is indicated. Clients may benefit from topical azelaic acid, topical metronidazole, or topical ivermectin and a low-dose oral antibiotic, like doxycycline (Consultant360, 2015). Client education should involve the use of moisturizer and sunscreen. Clients with persistent or difficult-to-manage symptoms should consult with a dermatologist.

SEBORRHEIC DERMATITIS

The adult client may present with chronic or relapsing sharply demarcated red, brown, or pink, greasy, scaly patches or plaques favoring the scalp, ears, face, central chest, and intertriginous areas. Management must include the periodic use of topical antifungal shampoos and creams, and rarely, oral antifungals such as fluconazole or itraconazole are required (Consultant360, 2015). The client with persistent or difficult-to-manage symptoms should be referred to a dermatologist for evaluation and management.

ECZEMA

The client with eczema may present to the primary care setting with acute, red, weeping, draining skin with blisters, or chronic, dry, thickened, scaly skin that is hyper- or depigmented. Etiologies may include irritants, allergies, or intrinsic causes, such as in the case of atopic eczema (Consultant360, 2015). Types include atopic dermatitis, contact dermatitis, stasis dermatitis, dyshidrotic eczema, seborrheic dermatitis, or asteatotic eczema.

Atopic dermatitis is one of the more common types. In children, pruritic, weeping, erythematous papules and plaques with some vesicles and crusting may appear on the cheeks, scalp, and extensor aspects of the extremities. In adults, more chronic, pruritic, licheni-fied plaques present on the hands or face (Consultant360, 2015). However, asteatotic eczema, or "winter's itch," commonly occurs in the elderly client who presents with dry, rough, scaly patches and plaques with superficial cracking of the skin on the shins, lower flanks, and posterior axillary line. The seasoned provider recom-mends the elimination of aggravating factors, such as frequent bath-ing, and the application of an emollient (Consultant360, 2015).

In the client with contact dermatitis, the priority for the skilled practitioner is to identify the causative substance and encourage avoidance. It has been reported that localized acute allergic contact dermatitis lesions may be treated with mid- to high-potency topical steroids, such as triamcinolone 0.1% (Kenalog, Aristocort) or clo-betasol 0.05% (Temovate). Thinner skinned regions of the body such as flexural surfaces, eyelids, face, and the anogenital region can be managed with lower-potency steroids, such as desonide ointment (Desowen). It has been further described that when the client's symp-toms involve more than 20% of the body surfaces, systemic steroid therapy is often required (Consultant360, 2015).

In general, if the symptoms of eczema are wet, the skillful practi-tioner is aware that the client needs drying agents such as water and aluminum acetate, and if they are dry, they need wetting agents such as ointments and creams. Topical therapies such as corticosteroids, immunosuppressives, or calcineurin inhibitors (tacrolimus oint-ment and pimecrolimus cream) are indicated, and systemic therapy is rarely necessary. Oral prednisone may be useful in some cases, and antibiotics may help when symptoms of secondary infection such as honey crusting become apparent (Consultant360, 2015). As always, the more difficult-to-manage client would benefit from a consulta-tion with a dermatologist. Client education includes the avoidance of triggers and liberal use of emollients within minutes of brief bathing with lukewarm-to-cooler water and moisturizing soaps.

PSORIASIS

The primary care client with psoriasis presents with lesions, which demonstrate sharply demarcated, scaly, erythematous plaques and occasional pustules. Initial management entails topical corticosteroids.

Ultraviolet light therapy may be indicated, and systemic agents can be considered if the client fails to respond to topical treatment. At this point, a referral to a specialist may be made. The skillful practitioner is aware that these clients may also complain of symptoms of psoriatic arthritis, and studies have indicated a higher risk of heart disease, obesity, type 2 diabetes, metabolic syndrome, and renal disease and to work up accordingly (Consultant360, 2015).

PITYRIASIS ROSEA

The client (most commonly aged 10–35 years) who presents with a rash that began as a large (4–10 cm) circular or oval spot on the chest, abdomen, or back (herald patch) followed by smaller spots that sweep out and resemble drooping pine tree branches will typically be diagnosed with pityriasis rosea. Symptoms may cause pruritis, are self-limiting, and usually go away within 10 weeks (Mayo Clinic, 2018). Effective management plans include oral or topical corticosteroids or oral antihistamines (American Academy of Family Physicians, 2019).

ALOPECIA

Management of the primary care client who presents with hair loss begins with a thorough history and focused examination. Information must be gathered regarding the duration, rate of progression, location, pattern, and extent of hair loss; associated symptoms; differentiation from breakage; hair care; and family history of hair loss.

Fast Facts

History guides the provider toward the appropriate etiology and type of alopecia. Examples include medications (e.g., colchicine, amantadine, amiodarone, anticoagulants, anticonvulsants, captopril, cholesterol-lowering drugs, cimetidine, hormones, isotretinoin, lithium, ketoconazole, propranolol, or valproic acid), poor diet, major illness or surgery, major psychological stress, significant weight loss, iron deficiency, weight loss, thyroid disorders, childbirth, or poisoning, and initial laboratory testing includes evaluation for thyroid disease as well as serum iron and ferritin to assess for iron deficiency (Shapiro, 2019).

As the management of alopecia is often complex, referral to a specialty provider to discuss and implement treatment options is appropriate.

WARTS

Clients will present to the primary care setting complaining of warts. Although there are many different types of warts, this section will focus on common and plantar warts. Other types of warts will typically be evaluated and managed by a dermatologist. The first-line treatment for common and plantar warts is topical salicylic acid and cryotherapy with liquid nitrogen, although plantar warts may be less likely to respond than common warts (Goldstein, Goldstein, & Morris-Jones, 2019).

Patient education is an integral part of the management of warts. Goldstein et al. (2019) report that salicylic acid is available in liquid, ointment, pad, and patch forms and is applied directly to the wart that is then covered by duct tape when the skin is dried daily and for no longer than 12 weeks. Furthermore, as cryotherapy is a clinician-administered treatment that may be painful, it should be reserved for adult clients and considered only when other therapies have been ineffective.

CELLULITIS/ABSCESS

Clients commonly report symptoms of skin infection to the primary care provider.

Management of skin and soft tissue infection depends on clinical presentation. For instance, clients with soft tissue skin infection, where there is an absence of drainable abscess or purulent drainage, should be managed with empiric antibiotic therapies only, such as penicillin, amoxicillin, cephalexin, clindamycin, or trimethoprim–sulfamethoxazole. Alternatively, the client with drainable abscess should undergo incision and drainage in addition to antibiotic therapy (Spelman & Baddour, 2019).

Coverage for methicillin-resistant *Staphylococcus aureus* (MRSA) should be considered in clients with a known history of MRSA infection, in the presence of a condition that increases risk, or who lack clinical response to agent that does not cover MRSA (Spelman & Baddour, 2019). The skillful provider obtains a wound culture when possible to determine that the empirical therapies prescribed are, in fact, appropriate for the management of skin and soft tissue infection. Parenteral therapies or referral for emergent care should be considered for more severe infection, such as in the presence of lymphangitis, streaking, or difficult-to-manage infections.

TINEAS

The client will often present with a fungal skin infection with a broad scope of clinical presentations on a variety of body sites. The lesion may commonly be a pruritic, circular or oval, or erythematous. Some may present as scaling patch, plaque, or erosions. Others spread centrifugally or have a central clearing. Tinea corporis (body), tinea pedis (feet), tinea cruris (groin), tinea faciei (face), and tinea manuum (hand) infections are typically superficial, involving only the epidermis, and can be managed with topical therapy with agents such as azoles, allylamines, butenafine, ciclopirox, and tolnaftate, and clients who require oral antifungal therapies are treated with terbinafine, itraconazole, or fluconazole (Goldstein & Goldstein, 2019). Tinea capitis (scalp) in the adult client is managed with oral terbinafine, itraconazole, fluconazole, or griseofulvin and tinea unguium (nail plate). Clients with onychomycosis, or any fungal nail infection, are managed using topical and systemic antifungal drugs, laser treatment, photodynamic therapy, or surgery (Goldstein & Bhatia, 2019). As fungal testing and/or liver function monitoring may be indicated, more severe or difficult-to-manage infections are typically referred to a specialist for management.

HERPES ZOSTER

The adult client who complains of a painful rash that initially presents as erythematous papules, typically in a single dermatome or several contiguous dermatomes, that progresses to grouped vesicles or bullae and then becomes pustular with or without systemic symptoms, such as headache, fever, malaise, or fatigue, will likely be diagnosed with herpes zoster. Risk factors include advancing age, immunocompromised status, the presence of autoimmune disease, and/or clients with a history of transplant (Albrecht & Levin, 2019).

Fast Facts

Antiviral therapy is recommended in clients with uncomplicated herpes zoster who present within 72 hours of clinical symptoms. Albrecht (2019) presents management recommendations that are provided as follows:

(continued)

(continued)

- Valacyclovir: 1,000 mg three times daily for 7 days
- Famciclovir: 500 mg three times daily for 7 days
- Acyclovir: 800 mg five times daily for 7 days

Antiviral therapy should reduce the pain associated with acute neuritis; however, the pain syndromes associated with herpes zoster can still be severe. Nonsteroidal anti-inflammatory drugs and acetaminophen should be recommended for mild pain, either alone or in combination with a weak opioid analgesic such as codeine or tramadol, and stronger opioid analgesic therapies such as oxycodone should be considered for moderate-to-severe pain (Albrecht, 2019). The client should be monitored for the effectiveness of the regimen and for the presence of a secondary bacterial infection. Recurrent or complicated infections should be referred to a specialist for evaluation and management.

IMPETIGO

Clients who present to the primary care practitioner complaining of localized lesions on the face or extremities that begin as papules and progress to vesicles surrounded by erythema that progress to form thick, adherent crusts with a golden appearance, in which systemic symptoms are usually absent and regional lymphadenitis may occur, are diagnosed with the condition nonbullous impetigo. Topical therapies (mupirocin or retapamulin) are to be recommended in clients who present with limited skin involvement, and oral therapies (cephalexin or dicloxacillin) are to be prescribed for clients with numerous lesions (Baddour, 2019).

SKIN CANCER SCREENING RECOMMENDATIONS

The skillful primary care provider plays an active role in client education regarding measures to prevent skin cancer and the importance of periodic screening. As it is not practical for every client to engage in screening by a dermatologist, the seasoned primary care practitioner must remain knowledgeable regarding principles of skin cancer assessment, as well as when it is more appropriate for the client to consult with a specialist. In general, using the guidelines presented in Table 5.2, suspicious lesions should be evaluated by a dermatologist (MedlinePlus, n.d.).

Table 5.2

Suspicious Lesions	
Asymmetry	The mole has an odd shape, with half of it not matching the other half
Border	The border of the mole is ragged or irregular
Color	The color of the mole is uneven
Diameter	The mole is bigger than the size of a pea or a pencil eraser
Evolution	The mole has changed in size, shape, or color

Fast Facts

- Mild acne does not require systemic therapy, yet moderate-to-severe symptoms likely require both topical and oral pharmacologic management.
- Clients with rosacea may benefit from topical azelaic acid, topical metronidazole, or topical ivermectin and a low-dose oral antibiotic, like doxycycline.
- Seborrheic dermatitis is typically managed with the periodic use of topical antifungal shampoos and creams, and rarely, oral antifungals such as fluconazole or itraconazole.
- Education for the client with eczema includes the avoidance of triggers and liberal use of emollients within minutes of brief bathing with lukewarm-to-cooler water and moisturizing soaps.
- Clients with psoriasis may also complain of symptoms of psoriatic arthritis, and these clients may have a higher risk of heart disease, obesity, type 2 diabetes, metabolic syndrome, and renal disease.
- Although self-limiting, pityriasis rosea can be managed effectively with oral or topical corticosteroids or oral antihistamines.
- The first-line treatment for common and plantar warts is topical salicylic acid and cryotherapy with liquid nitrogen.
- Clients with soft tissue skin infection, where there is an absence of drainable abscess or purulent drainage, should be managed with empiric antibiotic therapies only, such as penicillin, amoxicillin, cephalexin, clindamycin, or trimethoprim–sulfamethoxazole.
- Tinea infections are typically superficial, involving only the epidermis, and can be managed with topical therapy with agents.

(continued)

(*continued*)

- Risk factors for herpes zoster include advancing age, immunocompromised status, the presence of autoimmune disease, and/or clients with a history of transplant.
- Topical therapies are to be recommended for clients with impetigo who present with limited skin involvement, and oral therapies are to be prescribed for the client with numerous lesions.

SUMMARY

This journey through the subspecialties continued with a collaborative clinical practice session with physician specialists and nurse practitioners practicing in specialty settings. Clients presented with common dermatological complaints that often begin with their visit to the primary care provider. This clinical immersion experience led to the identification of conditions that the primary care provider is expected to diagnose or perhaps initiate during the management of clients with a variety of conditions affecting the skin. As always, effective management plans can only be developed once the provider has identified the correct etiology.

References

Albrecht, M. (2019). *Treatment of herpes zoster in the immunocompetent host*. UpToDate. Retrieved from https://www.uptodate.com/contents/treatment-of-herpes-zoster-in-the-immunocompetent-host

Albrecht, M., & Levin, M. (2019). *Epidemiology, clinical manifestations, and diagnosis of herpes zoster*. UpToDate. Retrieved from https://www.uptodate.com/contents/epidemiology-clinical-manifestations-and-diagnosis-of-herpes-zoster

American Academy of Family Physicians. (2019). *2019 AAFP FMX needs assessment*. Retrieved from https://www.aafp.org/dam/AAFP/documents/events/fmx/needs/fmx19-na-integ-dermatolotic-conditions.pdf

Baddour, L. (2019). *Impetigo*. UpToDate. Retrieved from https://www.uptodate.com/contents/impetigo?search=impetigo&source=search_result&selectedTitle=1~76&usage_type=default&display_rank=1

Consultant360. (2015). *Essentials of dermatology for the primary care provider*. Retrieved from https://www.consultant360.com/articles/essentials-dermatology-primary-care-provider

Goldstein, A., & Bhatia, N. (2019). *Onychomycosis: Management*. UpToDate. Retrieved from https://www.uptodate.com/contents/onychomycosis-management

Goldstein, A., & Goldstein, B. (2019). *Dermatophyte (tinea) infections.* UpToDate. Retrieved from https://www.uptodate.com/contents/dermatophyte-tinea -infections

Goldstein, B., Goldstein, A., & Morris-Jones, R. (2019). *Cutaneous warts (common, plantar, and flat warts).* UpToDate. Retrieved from https://www .uptodate.com/contents/cutaneous-warts-common-plantar-and-flat -warts?search=warts&source=search_result&selectedTitle=1~54&usage _type=default&display_rank=1

Mayo Clinic. (2018). *Pityriasis rosea.* Retrieved from https://www.mayoclinic .org/diseases-conditions/pityriasis-rosea/symptoms-causes/syc-20376405

MedlinePlus. (n.d.). *Skin cancer screening.* Retrieved from https://medlineplus .gov/lab-tests/skin-cancer-screening/

Shapiro, J. (2019). *Evaluation and diagnosis of hair loss.* UpToDate. Retrieved from https://www.uptodate.com/contents/evaluation-and-diagnosis-of -hair-loss?search=hair%20loss&source=search_result&selectedTitle=1~ 150&usage_type=default&display_rank=1

Spelman, D., & Baddour, L. (2019). *Cellulitis and skin abscess in adults: Treatment.* UpToDate. Retrieved from https://www.uptodate.com/contents/ cellulitis-and-skin-abscess-in-adults-treatment?search=cellulitis&source= search_result&selectedTitle=1~150&usage_type=default&display_rank=1

6

Practice Essentials for Endocrinology

At times, the client will present to primary care settings with hormonal complaints. It may, in fact, be the primary care provider who first diagnoses conditions related to the endocrine system. Common examples including those related to the thyroid gland, diabetes, weight management, and transgender health will be presented in this section. It is only through a thorough process of health history taking and the conduction of a comprehensive physical assessment that the skillful practitioner is effective in managing conditions related to the endocrine system and making a referral to a specialty provider when indicated.

THYROID

Hyperthyroidism

An excessive concentration of thyroid hormone may be caused by a variety of conditions. The most common causes of hyperthyroidism are Graves' disease, toxic multinodular goiter, toxic adenoma, or thyroiditis. Hyperthyroidism can be treated with antithyroid medications such as β-blockers to control adrenergic symptoms, methimazole or propylthiouracil, radioactive iodine ablation of the thyroid gland, or surgical thyroidectomy. The choice of treatment depends on the underlying diagnosis, presence of contraindications, severity, patient age, and patient preference (Kravets, 2016).

The clinical presentation of hyperthyroidism may range from asymptomatic to thyroid storm. Symptoms include palpitations, heat intolerance, diaphoresis, tremor, stare, lid lag, vitiligo, hyper-defecation, weight loss, anxiety, and insomnia. Chronic, untreated hyperthyroidism may result in atrial fibrillation or heart failure. The client undergoing estrogen, glucocorticoids, or dopamine therapy or the client who is pregnant or suffering from acute illness may present with abnormal thyroid function tests (Kravets, 2016).

Clinical suspicion of hyperthyroidism requires laboratory testing. The diagnostic workup for the client with hyperthyroidism includes the measurement of thyroid-stimulating hormone, free thyroxine (T4), and total triiodothyronine (T3) levels, radioactive iodine uptake unless contraindicated, and a scan of the thyroid gland (Kravets, 2016). The Endocrine Society/American Association of Clinical Endocrinologists does not recommend routinely ordering a thyroid ultrasound in patients with abnormal thyroid function tests with no palpable abnormality of the thyroid gland. Ultrasonography has been reported to be a cost-effective, safe alternative to radioactive iodine uptake and scanning (Kravets, 2016). It is often appropriate to refer the client with abnormal thyroid function testing to endocrinology to determine the proper workup and management plan.

Hypothyroidism

Hypothyroidism is commonly encountered in the primary care settings. The prevalence increases with age and is higher in female clients. It has been reported that, if left untreated, hypothyroidism can contribute to hypertension, dyslipidemia, infertility, cognitive impairment, and neuromuscular dysfunction (Gaitonde, 2012).

Autoimmune thyroid disease has been reported to be the most common cause of hypothyroidism in the United States. Symptomatology may be nonspecific and subtle, especially in older clients. The severity of the symptoms reflects the degree of dysfunction. Weight gain, fatigue, poor concentration, depression, diffuse muscle pain, coarse facies, and menstrual irregularities are symptoms of hypothyroidism. Additionally, symptoms with high specificity include constipation, cold intolerance, dry skin, proximal muscle weakness, and hair thinning or hair loss (Gaitonde, 2012).

Electrocardiography findings include bradycardia and flattened T-waves in clients with hypothyroidism. Patients with severe hypothyroidism may present with pericardial effusion, pleural effusion, megacolon, hemodynamic instability, and coma. Other laboratory findings in clients with hypothyroidism may include hyponatremia, hypercapnia, hypoxia, normocytic anemia, elevated creatine kinase, hyperprolactinemia, and hyperlipidemia (Gaitonde, 2012).

The best assessment of thyroid function is a serum thyroid-stimulating hormone, and no evidence suggests that screening asymptomatic adults improves outcomes. Symptom management can be accomplished through lifelong oral synthetic levothyroxine therapy. The starting dosage is 1.6 mcg per kg per day. Clients should be instructed to take thyroid hormone in the morning, 30 minutes before eating, avoiding calcium and iron supplements for 4 hours. Poor adherence is the most common cause of persistently uncontrolled hypothyroidism in clients on adequate doses of thyroid hormone. The dosage should be adjusted based on clinical response and follow-up laboratory testing (Gaitonde, 2012).

Older clients and those with known or suspected ischemic heart disease should be started on low-dose levothyroxine, rather than the full replacement dose, due to the risks of tachyarrhythmia or acute coronary syndrome. Pregnant clients often need their dosage increased. Drugs such as lithium, amiodarone, interferon alfa, interleukin-2, and tyrosine kinase inhibitors are associated with thyroid dysfunction. A number of medications can affect thyroid hormone levels such as sertraline, other selective serotonin reuptake inhibitors, tricyclic antidepressants, cholestyramine, carbamazepine, phenytoin, colestipol, orlistat, sucralfate, or estrogen-containing oral contraceptive or hormone therapy. The following are reasons to refer for endocrinology consultation: clients aged younger than 18 years or those with cardiac disease, coexisting endocrine diseases, suspected myxedema coma, pregnancy, presence of goiter, nodule, or other structural thyroid gland abnormality, or those who have been unresponsiveness to therapy (Gaitonde, 2012). A comparison of the symptoms of hyperthyroidism and hypothyroidism can be found in Table 6.1:

Table 6.1

Hyperthyroidism and Hypothyroidism Presentation	
Clinical Presentation of Hyperthyroidism	Clinical Presentation of Hypothyroidism
Palpitations	Weight gain
Heat intolerance	Fatigue
Diaphoresis	Poor concentration

(continued)

Table 6.1

Hyperthyroidism and Hypothyroidism Presentation (*continued*)

Clinical Presentation of Hyperthyroidism	Clinical Presentation of Hypothyroidism
Tremor	Depression
Stare	Diffuse muscle pain/proximal muscle weakness
Lid lag	Coarse facies
Vitiligo	Menstrual irregularities
Hyperdefecation	Hair thinning or hair loss
Weight loss	Constipation
Anxiety	Cold intolerance
Insomnia	Dry skin

Thyroid Nodules

Thyroid nodules are common in the general population, especially in women. Clients may present to primary care settings with symptoms of pressure in the neck, or a palpable mass may be discovered during physical examination. The risk of malignancy is small (Knox, 2013).

The measurement of thyroid-stimulating hormone can identify the condition, but ultrasonography and fine-needle aspiration are key elements of the diagnosis.

Fast Facts

A biopsy should be conducted for lesions larger than 1 cm and lesions with features suggestive of malignancy, and those in patients with risk factors for thyroid cancer (history of radiation to the head or neck especially in childhood) should be biopsied, regardless of size. Smaller lesions and those with benign histology can be followed and reevaluated.

The evaluation of thyroid nodules in euthyroid and hypothyroid pregnant women is the same as in other adults, and nodules in persons younger than 20 years or older than 70 years have an increased risk of malignancy (Knox, 2013).

If the pathology is malignant or suspicious for malignancy, surgery to remove the affected thyroid lobe or lobes is recommended so that a referral is indicated. Benign nodules should be followed with repeat ultrasonography 6 to 18 months after the initial fine-needle aspiration, and if the nodules have not grown significantly, a follow-up ultrasound may be extended to 3 to 5 years. If the nodule has grown, a repeat fine-needle aspiration should be performed (Knox, 2013).

DIABETES

It is well known that diabetes poses a significant financial burden on our healthcare system. It is, therefore, critical that the primary care provider is cognizant of the current guidelines and determines management plans in accordance with these standards. Diabetes should be managed by a multidisciplinary team that includes primary care physicians, subspecialty physicians, nurse practitioners, physician assistants, nurses, dietitians, exercise specialists, pharmacists, dentists, podiatrists, and mental health professionals (American Diabetes Association, 2019). Most often, a referral to an endocrinologist may be indicated. For the purpose of this chapter, the term diabetes refers to type 2 diabetes. The management of type 1, gestational, and other specific types of diabetes is beyond the scope and breadth of this book, as they are best managed by a specialty provider.

Diabetic testing for asymptomatic clients should be considered in adults of any age who are overweight or obese (body mass index [BMI] ≥ 25 kg/m^2 or ≥ 23 kg/m^2 in Asian Americans) and who have one or more additional risk factors for diabetes, and for all other clients, testing should begin at age 45 years. If tests are normal, repeat testing at a minimum of 3-year intervals. Monitoring for the development of type 2 diabetes in those with prediabetes (those whose glucose levels do not meet criteria for diabetes but are too high to be considered normal) should be done, at a minimum, annually (American Diabetes Association, 2019).

If a diagnosis of diabetes is made, an assessment of additional comorbid conditions should be conducted. Examples of conditions that affect diabetic management include atherosclerotic cardiovascular disease and heart failure; chronic kidney disease staging; hypertension; hyperlipidemia; cancers of the liver, pancreas, endometrium, colon/rectum, breast, and bladder; a history of cognitive impairment/dementia; nonalcoholic fatty liver disease; hepatocellular carcinoma; hearing impairment; psychosocial/emotional disorders; hip fractures; low testosterone in men; obstructive sleep apnea; and periodontal disease (American Diabetes Association, 2019).

The hemoglobin A1C is the primary measure studied in clinical trials demonstrating the benefits of improved glycemic control. A reasonable goal for the nonpregnant adult client is <7%. More stringent goals (<6.5%) may be reasonable in select patients, such as those with long life expectancies, if this can be achieved without significant hypoglycemia or other adverse effects. Less stringent A1C goals (<8%) may be appropriate for patients with a history of hypoglycemia (altered mental and/or physical state requiring assistance), limited life expectancies, advanced micro- or macrovascular complications, extensive comorbid conditions, or long-standing diabetes that has been difficult to manage (American Diabetes Association, 2019).

Self-monitoring of blood glucose may promote self-management and assist with medication adjustment decisions. Limited data suggest that continuous glucose monitoring may also be helpful in select patients, such as those on insulin. It is recommended that the A1C test be performed at least twice a year in patients who are meeting treatment goals and quarterly in patients whose medications have changed or in those who are not experiencing desired outcomes (American Diabetes Association, 2019).

Lifestyle intervention plays a critical role in diabetes and prediabetes management. For instance, an initial 7% loss of body weight and an increase in moderate-intensity physical activity to at least 150 minutes/week are recommended for clients with prediabetes. A low-calorie, low-fat eating plan should be encouraged with an emphasis on whole grains, legumes, nuts, fruits, and vegetables and minimal refined or processed foods. A referral to a nutritionist with expertise in diabetic management, such as the diabetes plate method, is often indicated. Diabetic patients can follow the same guidelines as those without diabetes if they choose to consume alcohol, and nonnutritive sweeteners may be an acceptable substitute when consumed in moderation. Smoking cessation counseling and other forms of treatment must also be routine components of the management of the diabetic client (American Diabetes Association, 2019).

The pharmacologic management of diabetes is an integral component of achieving optimal treatment outcomes. Metformin is the preferred initial pharmacologic agent for the diabetic client. It should also be considered in clients with prediabetes, especially for those with BMI ≥ 35 kg/m^2, aged <60 years, and women with a prior history of gestational diabetes mellitus. Once initiated, metformin should be continued as tolerated, and other agents, including insulin, can be added to achieve desired outcomes. Long-term use of metformin may be associated with vitamin B12 deficiency, so periodic measurement of vitamin B12 levels should be conducted, especially in those clients with anemia or peripheral neuropathy. The medication regimen should be reevaluated at regular intervals (every 3–6 months) and adjusted as needed (American Diabetes Association, 2019). Blood pressure and lipid management is an integral part of the management of the diabetic client (see Chapter 4, Practice Essentials for Cardiology).

Fast Facts

- In clients who have established cardiovascular disease, sodium–glucose cotransporter 2 inhibitors or glucagon-like peptide 1 receptor agonists are recommended.
- In clients with cardiovascular disease at high risk of heart failure or in whom heart failure coexists, sodium–glucose cotransporter 2 inhibitors are preferred.
- In clients with chronic kidney disease, consider use of a sodium–glucose cotransporter 2 inhibitors or glucagon-like peptide 1 receptor agonists to reduce risk of progression and/or cardiovascular events (American Diabetes Association, 2019).

Glucagon should be prescribed for clients at increased risk of hypoglycemia. Caregivers or family members of these individuals should know where it is and when and how to administer as glucagon administration is not limited to the healthcare professional. One or more episodes of hypoglycemia should trigger a reevaluation of the treatment regimen (American Diabetes Association, 2019).

Diabetes technology, or the hardware, devices, and software to administer insulin and monitor blood glucose, is constantly changing. When applied appropriately, this technology can improve the lives and health of people with diabetes (American Diabetes Association, 2019). The provider must remain current on technological advances in diabetic management and supply the client with the tools available to achieve optimal treatment options.

Diabetic management principles vary in the presence of select conditions. For example, diabetic clients with chronic kidney disease and/or comorbid hypertension require an annual assessment of urinary albumin and estimated glomerular filtration rate (eGFR). The optimization of glucose and blood pressure control is to be encouraged to slow kidney disease progression. Metformin is contraindicated in patients with an eGFR <30 mL, and eGFR should be monitored while taking metformin. In nonpregnant patients with diabetes and hypertension, either an angiotensin-converting enzyme (ACE) inhibitor or an angiotensin receptor blocker (ARB) is recommended. The skillful provider is certain to monitor serum creatinine and potassium levels when ACE inhibitors, ARBs, or diuretics are used. An ACE inhibitor or ARB is not recommended for the primary prevention of chronic kidney disease in patients with diabetes who have normal blood pressure, normal urinary albumin-to-creatinine ratio, and normal eGFR. Prompt referral to a specialty provider is indicated with uncertainty about the etiology of kidney disease, difficult management issues, and rapidly progressing kidney disease (American Diabetes Association, 2019).

Diabetic clients should have a comprehensive eye examination by an ophthalmologist at the time of the diagnosis. Glycemic control is to be optimized in order to reduce the risk or slow the progression of diabetic retinopathy. Without evidence of retinopathy for one or more annual eye exams and with glycemia in good control, subsequent exams every 1 to 2 years are sufficient (American Diabetes Association, 2019).

Diabetic clients are to be assessed for peripheral neuropathy upon diagnosis and again annually. It has been reported that neuropathic pain can impact quality of life, limit mobility, and contribute to depression and/or social dysfunction. Therefore, the optimization of glucose control to prevent, delay, or slow the progression of the neuropathy is indicated. Pregabalin, duloxetine, and gabapentin are to be considered as the initial pharmacologic options for neuropathic pain. An annual assessment of the feet and education on preventative foot care is critical (American Diabetes Association, 2019).

The latest recommendations include that providers incorporate an assessment of social context, including food insecurity, housing stability, and financial barriers, and apply this information into the plan of care. Self-management support and referral to community resources are important components to the reduction of health disparities and the overall management of diabetes (American Diabetes Association, 2019). The seasoned provider completes a comprehensive assessment of social needs to reduce health disparities and promote optimal care of the diabetic client.

WEIGHT MANAGEMENT

Weight management is an important facet of primary care practice. Elements of the effects of obesity are presented in Chapter 4, Practice Essentials for Cardiology, and Chapter 16, Practice Essentials for

Pediatrics. This chapter focuses on the role of hormones in the obese client and related strategies to promote weight management.

Appetite-related hormones play a role in weight regain after weight loss and following weight loss as a result of dieting; it has been demonstrated that there are increased levels of ghrelin and gastric inhibitory polypeptide with decreased levels of leptin, peptide YY, cholecystokinin, amylin, insulin, and glucagon-like peptide 1. Alterations in these hormones result in weight regain by increasing hunger (Greenway, 2015). Therefore, the client needs to be educated not only on strategies to promote healthy weight loss and the maintenance of a healthy body weight but also on the risk of and rationale for weight regain following weight loss, as well as the strategies to promote long-term weight loss.

Lifestyle modification, the key to weight management, consists of a combination of diet, physical activity, and behavior therapy. Weight loss medication has been proven to facilitate adherence, reduce hunger, increase satiation, and/or block the absorption of nutrients. Adding medication to lifestyle counseling increases weight loss as compared with counseling alone (Wadden et al., 2013). Table 6.2 is a summary of the current pharmacological options for weight loss.

Table 6.2

Medications for Weight Loss

Weight Loss Medication	How It Works	Common Side Effects	Warnings
Orlistat (Xenical) Available in lower dose without prescription (Alli)	Works in the gut to reduce the amount of fat absorption.	Diarrhea Gas Leakage of oily stools Stomach pain	Rare cases of severe liver injury have been reported. Avoid taking with cyclosporine. Recommend taking with multivitamins.
Lorcaserin (Belviq)	Acts on the serotonin receptors in the brain resulting in the feeling of fullness after eating smaller amounts of food.	Constipation Cough Dizziness Dry mouth Feeling tired Headaches Nausea	Tell your doctor if you take antidepressants or migraine medications, as some of these can cause problems when taken together.

(continued)

Table 6.2

Medications for Weight Loss (*continued*)

Weight Loss Medication	How It Works	Common Side Effects	Warnings
Phentermine–topiramate (Qsymia)	Phentermine lessens appetite, and topiramate is used to treat seizures or migraine headaches. Reduces hunger or makes one feel full sooner.	Constipation Dizziness Dry mouth Taste changes, especially with carbonated beverages Tingling of your hands and feet Trouble sleeping	Do not use in clients with glaucoma or hyperthyroidism or those with a history of heart attack or stroke, abnormal heart rhythm, kidney disease, or mood problems. As it may lead to birth defects, do not prescribe to clients who are pregnant or planning a pregnancy, or to breastfeeding clients.
Naltrexone–bupropion (Contrave)	Naltrexone is used to treat alcohol and drug dependence, and bupropion is used to treat depression. Reduces hunger or makes one feel full sooner.	Constipation Diarrhea Dizziness Dry mouth Headache Increased blood pressure Increased heart rate Insomnia Liver damage Nausea/vomiting	Do not use in clients with uncontrolled high blood pressure, seizures, or a history of anorexia or bulimia nervosa. Avoid in clients who are dependent on opioid pain medications or withdrawing from drugs or alcohol. May increase suicidal thoughts or actions.
Liraglutide (Saxenda) Available by injection only	Reduces hunger or makes one feel full sooner. Under a different name, Victoza, approved to treat type 2 diabetes.	Nausea Diarrhea Constipation Abdominal pain Headache Raised pulse	May increase the chance of developing pancreatitis. Has been found to cause a rare type of thyroid tumor in animals.

(*continued*)

Table 6.2

Medications for Weight Loss (*continued*)			
Weight Loss Medication	**How It Works**	**Common Side Effects**	**Warnings**
Other medications to curb desire to eat include the following: Phentermine Benzphetamine Diethylpropion Phendimetrazine	Increase chemicals in the brain to make one feel that they are not hungry or that they are full. **Note**: FDA-approved only for short-term use—up to 12 weeks.	Dry mouth Constipation Difficulty sleeping Dizziness Feeling nervous Feeling restless Headache Raised blood pressure Raised pulse	Do not use in clients with heart disease, uncontrolled high blood pressure, hyperthyroidism, or glaucoma. Avoid in clients with severe anxiety or other mental health problems.

FDA, Food and Drug Administration.

Source: National Institute of Diabetes and Digestive and Kidney Diseases. (2016). *Prescription medications to treat overweight and obesity: What are overweight and obesity?* Retrieved from https://www.niddk.nih.gov/health-information/ weight-management/prescription-medications-treat-overweight-obesity

TRANSGENDER MEDICINE

The management of transgender health needs is an important component of primary care practice. Although the practice of gender transition involves a team approach consisting of experts from endocrinology, psychology, surgery, and other members of the gender health team, transgender clients may present to primary care settings seeking primary care services, so the skillful practitioner must be knowledgeable and competent. Transgender refers to a person whose gender identity differs from the sex that was assigned at birth, and transsexual refers to an individual who has sought medical intervention to transition to their identified gender (Hashemi, Weinreb, Weimer, & Weiss, 2018).

Fast Facts

The International Statistical Classification of Diseases and Related Health Problems, 10th Revision, criteria for transsexualism include the following:

(continued)

(*continued*)

- The desire to live and be accepted as a member of the opposite sex, usually accompanied by the wish to make their body as congruent as possible with the preferred sex through surgery and hormone treatment.
- The transsexual identity has been present persistently for at least 2 years.
- The disorder is not a symptom for another mental disorder, genetic disorder, disorder of sex development, or chromosomal abnormality (Hashemi et al., 2018).

Sexual orientation describes sexual attraction only and is not related to gender identity, and gender dysphoria refers to distress experienced when one's gender identity and sex are not completely congruent. Transgender clients may avoid seeking care due to negative experiences or fear. Preferred name and pronouns should be documented in the electronic health record for all providers and staff (Hashemi et al., 2018). All members of the healthcare team, including staff, must use the terminology correctly and be sensitive to the client's unique healthcare needs in the provision of effective, high-quality, culturally competent care.

The provider should examine and obtain information that focuses solely on the issues for which the client is seeking care for. For instance, a physical exam of the chest and genitals may be distressing to the client. If indicated, the provider and patient should have a discussion on its importance and plan to optimize the patient's comfort (Hashemi et al., 2018).

Screening is an integral role of primary care practice. As breast cancer may be a concern in transgender women due to prolonged estrogen exposure, the seasoned provider is knowledgeable and applies the current standards related to breast cancer screening. Male-to-female individuals who have known increased risk should follow screening recommendations for nontransgender women if they are aged 50 years or older and have had more than 5 years of hormone use, and for female-to-male clients who have not had chest surgery, screening guidelines should follow those for nontransgender women. Guidelines for those who have had chest reconstruction do not exist, and mammography may be difficult so chest wall examination, MRI, and/or ultrasound may be indicated (Hashemi et al., 2018).

Prostate cancer screening is recommended in transgender women as per standard guidelines; however, because the prostate-specific antigen level is expected to be reduced due to hormonal therapy, a reading over 1.0 is considered abnormal. Cervical cancer screening is conducted in transgender men; samples must note the site (cervical and not anal), and it is important to document whether the client receives testosterone therapy and has amenorrhea. Following vaginoplasty, a pap is not indicated as transgender women do not have a cervix (Hashemi et al., 2018). Sexually transmitted infection assessment should be based on current anatomy and sexual behaviors. The effect of hormonal treatment on cardiovascular health remains controversial in the literature, so risk calculation and use of aspirin and/or statin therapy should be considered based on age, race, gender, and other risk factors. Finally, transgender women who use cross-sex hormonal therapies may be at increased risk for venous thromboembolism and should be evaluated when presenting with relevant symptomatology (Hashemi et al., 2018).

Fast Facts

- Symptoms to observe for in the client with hyperthyroidism include palpitations, heat intolerance, diaphoresis, tremor, stare, lid lag, vitiligo, hyperdefecation, weight loss, anxiety, and insomnia.
- Refer endocrinology consultation to clients with hypothyroidism and aged younger than 18 years or those with cardiac disease, coexisting endocrine diseases, suspected myxedema coma, pregnancy, presence of goiter, nodule, or other structural thyroid gland abnormality, or those who have been unresponsiveness to therapy.
- The provider must incorporate an assessment of social context, including food insecurity, housing stability, and financial barriers, and apply this information into the plan of care of the diabetic client.
- All members of the healthcare team, including staff, must use the terminology correctly and be sensitive to the transgender client's unique healthcare needs in the provision of effective, high-quality, culturally competent care.
- Adding weight loss medication to lifestyle counseling increases weight loss as compared with counseling alone.

SUMMARY

This journey through the subspecialties continued with a variety of collaborative clinical practice sessions with physician specialists and nurse practitioners practicing in specialty settings. Clients presented with common endocrinological/hormonal complaints that often begin with their visit to the primary care provider. This clinical immersion experience led to the identification of hot topics that the primary/urgent care nurse practitioner is expected to diagnose or perhaps initiate management of. As always, effective management plans can only be developed once the provider has identified the correct etiology.

References

American Diabetes Association. (2019). Standards of medical care in diabetes—2019 abridged for primary care providers. *Clinical Diabetes, 37*(1), 11–34. doi:10.2337/cd18-0105

Gaitonde, D. (2012). Hypothyroidism: An update. *American Family Physician, 86*(3), 244–251.

Greenway, F. (2015). Physiological adaptations to weight loss and factors favoring weight regain. *International Journal of Obesity, 39*, 1188–1196. doi:10.1038/ijo.2015.59

Hashemi, L., Weinreb, J., Weimer, A., & Weiss, R. (2018). Transgender care in the primary care setting: A review of guidelines and literature. *Federal Practitioner, 38*(7), 30–37.

Knox, M. (2013). Thyroid nodules. *American Family Physician, 88*(3), 193–196.

Kravets, I. (2016). Hyperthyroidism: Diagnosis and treatment. *American Family Physician, 93*(5), 363–370.

National Institute of Diabetes and Digestive and Kidney Diseases. (2016). *Prescription medications to treat overweight and obesity: What are overweight and obesity?* Retrieved from https://www.niddk.nih.gov/health-information/weight-management/prescription-medications-treat-overweight-obesity

Wadden, T., Volger, S., Tsai, A., Sarwer, D., Berkowitz, R., Diewald, L., &Vetter, M. (2013). Managing obesity in primary care practice: An overview and perspective from the POWER-UP study. *International Journal of Obesity, 37*(1), S3–S11. doi:10.1038/ijo.2013.90

7

Practice Essentials for Gastroenterology

This journey through the subspecialties continues with some of the most common complaints that result in the client's visit to the primary care provider—disorders of the gastrointestinal system. Although these conditions can originate in a variety of sites, many begin at or involve the stomach. The stomach is like the rug at the entrance of the house. It takes the most wear and tear (Brelvi, 2019). Damage may result due to increased acid production and/or the consumption of certain foods, alcohol, caffeine, and medication(s). As always, management plans can only be developed once the provider has identified the source and the location of the damage.

ABDOMINAL PAIN

A client may present to primary care settings with abdominal pain. In most primary/urgent care settings where nurse practitioners (NPs) practice, access to immediate diagnostic testing results may be limited. It is the role of the skillful diagnostician to first rule out any acute medical or surgical emergency. Some examples of medical or surgical emergencies are provided in Box 7.1.

It is important to note that if a medical or surgical emergency is expected, referral to the nearest emergency department is indicated.

Spleen

Although the spleen is actually a part of the lymphatic system, its location in the left upper quadrant of the abdomen leads to its

BOX 7.1 EXAMPLE MEDICAL OR SURGICAL EMERGENCIES

- Appendicitis
- Abdominal aortic aneurysm
- Ectopic pregnancy
- Renal calculi
- Ruptured ovarian cysts
- Cholelithiasis
- Pelvic inflammatory disease

mention here. The patient who presents to the primary/urgent care setting with splenomegaly, pain or fullness in the left upper abdomen or left shoulder that worsens on taking a deep breath, feeling full without eating or eating a small amount, anemia, fatigue, frequent infections, or easy bleeding requires further evaluation. Rupture is a potential complication of an enlarged spleen. Initial diagnostics include blood work and an ultrasound, and a referral to a specialty provider for a bone marrow biopsy may also be indicated (Landaw et al., 2016).

Gallbladder

Pain may also occur in the lower or upper right abdomen spreading to the right upper back or shoulder blade, which may indicate cholelithiasis. Other common symptoms include vomiting, right upper quadrant tenderness, and a low-grade fever. Symptoms can increase in severity when a stone blocks a portion of, or the entire, biliary tract. After symptom assessment, abdominal ultrasound generally confirms diagnosis (Thomson, Shaffer, & Gonska, 2013).

Fast Facts

Although extremely rare, gallbladder cancer presents with symptoms similar to gallstone disease, such as nausea, vomiting, pain, and anorexia. The highest risk is for patients with symptomatic gallbladder disease, and surgery is the only curative treatment for this type of cancer (British Columbia Cancer Agency, 2009).

Gallbladder polyps can be associated with gallbladder cancer. Larger polyps (>10 mm) are more likely to be malignant or will become cancerous over time (Andersson & Friedman, 2016). Genetics increase a client's risk for malignancy.

Pancreas

The patient may also present with pain in the upper abdomen or back with nausea. This can result from acute pancreatitis. The most common cause of acute pancreatitis is gallstones. Alcohol abuse is the second most common cause, which can lead to chronic pancreatitis. Chronic pancreatitis may affect insulin production, potentially leading to diabetes. An abdominal CT scan or ultrasound aids in diagnosis. Amylase levels may be increased but are less reliable with chronic pancreatitis than with acute. Patients with a history of excess alcohol use must completely stop consuming it to slow further disease progression (LaRusch, Solomon, & Whitcomb, 2014).

It is imperative that the NP be mindful that pancreatic cancer is the third leading cause of cancer death in the United States. Signs of pancreatic cancer that are monitored include abdominal/back pain, ascites, loss of appetite, nausea, indigestion, weight loss, jaundice, change in stools, and new onset or change in diabetic control. Risk factors include family history, diet, obesity, race, smoking, gender, age, and history of diabetes and/or pancreatitis (AskMayoExpert, 2015). As always, the NP can play an integral role in diagnosis, patient education, and prompt referral.

Initiating Diagnostic Testing

Of course, abdominal pain may also result from acute infection such as cystitis or chronic conditions such as gastritis or gastric ulcer. Regardless of whether the source of the pain is acute or chronic, it is likely that a specialty provider such as a surgeon or gastroenterologist will need to be consulted and the patient transitioned into their care. In today's complex healthcare system, there are often delays until these consultation(s) may be approved, scheduled, and actually take place. Therefore, the primary care provider is often left to initiate the diagnostic workup. Blood work and/or urine studies may, of course, be indicated. At times, an x-ray or ultrasound is an appropriate first step, as they are noninvasive and relatively inexpensive. Additional imaging such as an MRI or CT scan may also be indicated. Regardless, there are a number of hot topics that today's primary care provider must consider to initiate diagnosis and proceed with management planning when indicated and appropriate.

CHANGES IN THE STOOL

Whether accompanied by abdominal pain or not, it is typical for a patient to present to primary and/or urgent care settings complaining of changes in the stool. Constipation, diarrhea (acute or chronic), flatulence, blood in the stool, or changes in the stool should be considered significant and evaluated appropriately. Standard guidelines exist, of course, regarding indications to initiate and repeat colonoscopy based on age, family history, and previous presence of polyps, small bowel, or colonic disease.

Fast Facts

Diet, obesity, smoking, and genetic predisposition are potential risk factors for colorectal disease. Research is currently underway investigating the role of microbiota and its effect on the gut—a hot topic in gastroenterology today.

Microbiota

Microorganisms live inside the gastrointestinal tract, and we all have our own unique microbiota (MacGill, 2018). These play an important role in absorption, digestion, immunity, and behavior and may be linked to a number of diseases. Bacterial populations are being explored in conditions such as inflammatory bowel diseases, irritable bowel syndrome, vitamin deficiencies such as vitamin D, obesity, and type 2 diabetes (MacGill, 2018). Discoveries are being made to help identify ways to limit the invasion of potentially harmful microbes and their disease-causing effects so that the identification and management of gut microbiota are becoming a cornerstone of preventive medicine (MacGill, 2018). Foods containing probiotics or probiotic supplementation may restore the composition of the gut, introducing beneficial functions to gut microbial communities, resulting in amelioration or prevention of gut inflammation and other intestinal diseases (Hemarajata & Versalovic, 2013).

FROM NAUSEA TO NUTRITION

A number of other common gastrointestinal symptoms lead patients to visit the primary care provider. Nausea, vomiting, dyspepsia (indigestion), belching, bloating, and heartburn may signify a variety of esophageal or gastric conditions for the NP to evaluate. Depending on the duration and severity of the condition, often a specialty provider will be consulted or the patient will be transferred to the care of a specialist. Yet, the NP is often responsible for the initial evaluation and corresponding workup to determine whether further assessment via endoscopy is indicated. The management of these common conditions presents an additional hot topic in the field of gastroenterology.

Gastroesophageal Reflux Disease

Gastroesophageal reflux disease (GERD), intermittent gastroesophageal (acid) reflux and its symptoms that occur regularly and/or interfere with daily life, , is caused by a multitude of well-known etiologies. Obesity, pregnancy, presence of a hiatal hernia, and other dietary and lifestyle choices are some common offenders. Lifestyle modification, pharmacologic management, surgical intervention, and endoluminal therapies are today's treatment options for the patient with GERD, and although not all patients are candidates for invasive interventions, concerns over the side effects of long-term use of proton pump inhibitors such as dementia (controversial and not evidence-based), osteoporosis, chronic kidney dysfunction, electrolyte imbalances, pneumonia, and *Clostridium difficile* infection have directed patients and providers to consider nonpharmacologic approaches (Sandhu & Fass, 2018).

Polat and Polat (2012) report that GERD has a multifactorial etiology. However, the nature of the relationship between *Helicobacter pylori* (HP) infection and reflux esophagitis remains unclear. A 3-year study of 2,442 patients was conducted to find the influence of HP on GERD. Results included that HP positive was frequently seen in patients with GERD. In addition, a statistically significant relationship was found between HP positivity and the grade of GERD. Furthermore, HP infection was found in 82.5% of patients with GERD. Controversy still exists about the association between GERD and HP infection. Based on these findings, significant evidence suggests the potential role of HP infection in the development of GERD, as the data provide sufficient evidence to define the relationship between GERD and HP infection (Polat & Polat, 2012).

Furthermore, evidence suggests that stress reduction is an additional recognized lifestyle modification for the NP to consider in GERD management. In a study of over 12,000 patients with GERD, "feelings of continued stress" was the most common lifestyle factor (45.6% of patients) reported (Haruma et al., 2015). It is, therefore, the role of the NP to gather a thorough and comprehensive history and educate the client on stress reduction and other lifestyle changes and their role in controlling the symptoms of GERD. A referral to a nutritionist, psychologist, or other members of the interdisciplinary team may, in fact, be indicated for the management of GERD symptoms related to lifestyle in collaboration with the gastroenterologist, surgeon, or other related specialty providers.

LIVER

Beyond the gastrointestinal tract, conditions related to the liver pose some additional hot topics for the primary care NP to explore and understand.

Fast Facts

Important elements that the skillful practitioner is careful to consider in the comprehensive health history related to conditions affecting the liver include, but are not limited to:

- International travel
- Alcohol intake
- Diet
- Exercise
- Family history
- Bowel habits
- Joint pain
- Fatigue

Liver function testing (LFT) is an inexpensive diagnostic aid to determine if a patient's symptomatology is related to the liver. In general, increased LFTs result from hepatitis B/C, chemical injury (medications such as acetaminophen), autoimmune etiology, or a storage problem.

Fatty Liver

Fatty liver is becoming more and more common. Currently, 30 to 60 million individuals in the United States are affected. Some estimates are even greater. Fatty liver results from a storage problem, where excess calories are taken in and not used. A comparison can be made to excess funds stored in a bank account and not spent (Brelvi, 2019). The body does not reject these additional calories, so they are stored in the liver. Treatment involves a low-calorie diet as fewer calories and less fat will lead to the creation of more space. The initial goal should be to reduce body weight by 10%. Furthermore, exercise and supplementation, such as omega-3 fish oil, vitamin E, and lecithin, are recommended to protect liver cells. Increased copper and iron levels may be found in these patients. Ongoing monitoring is included in the management of patients with fatty liver.

Hepatitis

Although hepatitis B is a potentially life-threatening liver condition, a vaccine that is 95% effective has been available since 1982. A total of 2,967 cases of acute hepatitis C virus (HCV) were reported from 42 states in 2016, where the overall incidence rate was 1.0 cases per 100,000 population, an increase from 2015 (0.8 cases per 100,000 population; Centers for Disease Control and Prevention, n.d.). Therefore, HCV screening is recommended for clients aged 45 to 65 years so that diagnosis and referral for management may be initiated in primary care settings. Mahadevan (2017) reports that the management of HCV, after the cure, is achievable in over 95% of patients resulting in a sharp decline in the need for liver transplant. Patients at risk for reinfection should have HCV RNA testing annually or if their liver enzymes increase. If pretreatment fibrosis is low, no further monitoring is needed, and they can follow up with their primary care provider. Modifiable risk factors, such as metabolic fatty liver and alcohol abuse, should be identified with appropriate counseling provided (Mahadevan, 2017). These are the important screening guidelines and interventions for the NP in primary care to consider and incorporate into management plans.

HEMORRHOIDS

Hemorrhoids, or piles, are swollen veins in the anus and lower rectum resulting from straining during a bowel movement (BM) or from the increased pressure during pregnancy. Hemorrhoids may be internal or external. Hemorrhoids are very common and, therefore, often result in a patient's visit to primary and/or urgent care settings. Symptoms include itching, discomfort, and bleeding. Occasionally, a clot may form. These thrombosed hemorrhoids are not dangerous but can be extremely painful and sometimes need to be lanced and drained. Whether present or not, it is not safe to assume that rectal bleeding is due to the hemorrhoid. As rectal bleeding can occur with other diseases and can be a warning sign for colorectal cancer, the primary care provider must direct the patient to the appropriate specialty provider for evaluation and management. Furthermore, emergency care may be indicated with large amounts of rectal bleeding, lightheadedness, or faintness (Jacobs, 2014).

Rectal Prolapse

Finally, it is important to rule out a rectal prolapse before making the diagnosis of a hemorrhoid. Here, Meher (2016) describes how symptoms may include an awareness of protrusion upon wiping, inability to control BMs, loss of urge to defecate, mucus or blood discharge, and/or pain during BMs. A rectal prolapse usually has circular folds, whereas an internal hemorrhoid has radial folds (Meher, 2016). A specialist will likely be consulted when there is possible presence of a rectal prolapse as treatment involves surgery.

Fast Facts

- If abdominal pain is severe and a medical or surgical emergency is expected, referral to the nearest emergency department is indicated.
- Changes in the stool should be considered significant until proven otherwise and evaluated appropriately.
- Stress reduction and other recognized lifestyle modifications are to be considered in GERD management.
- Fatty liver results from a storage problem, where excess calories are taken in and not used.
- HCV screening is recommended for all clients aged 45 to 65 years.
- Whether present or not, it is not safe to assume that rectal bleeding is due to a hemorrhoid.

SUMMARY

This journey through the subspecialties continued with a variety of collaborative clinical practice sessions with physician specialists and NPs practicing in specialty settings. Patients presented with common complaints that often begin with their visit to the primary care provider. This clinical immersion experience led to the identification of hot topics that the primary/urgent care NP is expected to diagnose or perhaps initiate management as they relate to the gastrointestinal system. As always, effective management plans can only be developed once the provider has identified the correct etiology.

References

Andersson, K. L., & Friedman, L. S. (2016). Acalculous biliary pain, acute acalculous cholecystitis, cholesterolosis, adenomyomatosis, and gallbladder polyps. In M. Feldman, L. S. Friedman, & L. J. Brandt (Eds.), *Sleisenger and Fordtran's gastrointestinal and liver disease: Pathophysiology, diagnosis, management* (10th ed.). Philadelphia, PA: Saunders Elsevier.

AskMayoExpert. (2015). *Pancreatic cancer.* Rochester, MN.: Mayo Foundation for Medical Education and Research.

Brelvi, Z. (2019). *Collaborative clinical practice sessions.* Bloomfield, NJ.

British Columbia Cancer Agency. (2009). *Gastrointestinal cancer management guidelines, gallbladder.* Retrieved from http://www.bccancer.bc.ca/health-professionals/clinical-resources/cancer-management-guidelines/gastrointestinal/gallbladder

Centers for Disease Control and Prevention. (n.d.). *Hepatitis C.* Retrieved from https://www.cdc.gov/hepatitis/hcv/index.htm

Haruma, K., Kinoshinta, Y., Sakamoto, S., Sanada, K., Hiroi, S., & Miwa, H. (2015). Lifestyle factors and efficacy of lifestyle interventions in gastroesophageal reflux disease patients with functional dyspepsia: Primary care perspectives from the LEGEND study. *Internal Medicine, 54*(7), 695–701. doi:10.2169/internalmedicine.54.3056

Hemarajata, P., & Versalovic, J. (2013). Effects of probiotics on gut microbiota: Mechanisms of intestinal immunomodulation and neuromodulation. *Therapeutic Advances in Gastroenterology, 6*(1), 39–51. doi:10.1177/1756283X12459294

Jacobs, D. (2014). Hemorrhoids. *New England Journal of Medicine, 371*, 944–951. doi:10.1056/NEJMcp1204188

Landaw, S., et al. (2016). *Approach to the adult patient with splenomegaly and other splenic disorders.* Retrieved from https://www.uptodate.com/contents/evaluation-of-splenomegaly-and-other-splenic-disorders-in-adults

LaRusch, J., Solomon, S., & Whitcomb, D. (2014). *Pancreatitis overview.* Retrieved from https://www.ncbi.nlm.nih.gov/books/NBK190101/

MacGill, M. (2018). What are the gut microbiota and human microbiome? *Medical News Today,* Retrieved from https://www.medicalnewstoday.com/articles/307998.php

Mahadevan, U. (2017). *Conference coverage: Hot topics in 2017.* Retrieved from https://www.mdedge.com/gihepnews/article/145344/liver-disease/hot-topics-2017

Meher, S. (2016). Complete rectal prolapse vs prolapsed hemorrhoids: Points to ponder. *Pan African Medical Journal, 24,* 88. doi:10.11604/pamj.2016.24.88.9760

Polat, F., & Polat, S. (2012). The effect of *Helicobacter pylori* on gastroesophageal reflux disease. *JSLS, 16*(2), 260–263. doi:10.4293/108680812X13427982376860

Sandhu, D., & Fass, R. (2018). Current trends in the management of gastro-esophageal reflux disease. *Gut Liver, 12*(1), 7–16. doi:10.5009/gnl16615

Thomson, A., Shaffer, E., & Gonska, T. (2013). The biliary system. In A. Thomson & E. Shaffer (Eds.), *First principles of gastroenterology: The basis of disease and approach to management* (7th ed.). Mississauga, ON: AstraZeneca Canada Inc.

8

Practice Essentials for Hematology and Oncology

The adult client may present to the primary care setting with a variety of symptoms related to hematology and/or oncology. Although many of these are appropriate for the primary care provider to diagnose and manage, some conditions may be persistent or significant enough to be referred to the hematologist or oncologist. The skillful provider is knowledgeable on the standards of care for the client with a hematological–oncological condition, as well as the red flags to assess and refer for a consultation with the correct specialty provider. The primary care management of the client with a history of cancer is also presented in this chapter.

MANAGEMENT OF SELECT HEMATOLOGIC CONDITIONS IN PRIMARY CARE

Bleeding and Bruising

Clients may report easy bruising and abnormal bleeding in the primary care setting. Examples include excessive bruising when injured, epistaxis, menorrhagia, or prolonged bleeding following dental procedures. A thorough history including medication review and family history is an important component of initial management. Select antibiotics such as cephalosporins, linezolid, nitrofurantoin, penicillin, rifampin, sulfonamides, and vancomycin may result in symptoms of bruising or bleeding. Other examples of medications that may result in these symptoms are provided by Neutze and Roque (2016) and are presented in Box 8.1.

BOX 8.1 MEDICATIONS THAT MAY RESULT IN BLEEDING AND BRUISING

Alcohol	Dabigatran	Rivaroxaban
Apixaban	Enoxaparin	Select antibiotics
Aspirin	Fish oil	SSRIs
Carbamazepine	Heparin	Thiazide diuretics
Clopidogrel	NSAIDs	Valproic acid
Corticosteroids	Quinine	Warfarin

NSAID, nonsteroidal anti-inflammatory drug; SSRI, selective serotonin reuptake inhibitor.

Source: Data from Neutze, D., & Roque, J. (2016). Clinical evaluation of bleeding and bruising in primary care. *American Family Physician, 93*(4), 279–286.

Furthermore, a history of physical abuse must be considered and excluded. Upon comprehensive physical examination, it has been reported that a clinical finding of mucocutaneous bleeding may suggest platelet dysfunction, and hemarthroses or hematomas are more common in coagulopathies (Neutze & Roque, 2016).

The diagnostic workup of the client with abnormal bruising and bleeding includes a complete blood count, peripheral blood smear, prothrombin time (PT), and partial thromboplastin time (PTT). Neutze and Roque (2016) go on to describe a number of possible conditions related to bruising and bleeding. For instance, a normal PT/PTT indicates a platelet disorder such as von Willebrand disease; a mixing study should be performed with a normal PT/prolonged PTT; a vitamin K challenge is indicated with an abnormal PT/ normal PTT; and a workup for liver failure is warranted with prolonged PT/PTT. As always, the skillful primary care practitioner is certain to refer the client to a hematologist when a consultation with a specialty provider for further evaluation and management of the client with abnormal bruising and bleeding is indicated.

Anemia

The primary care provider is often faced with the evaluation and management of the client with anemia. At times, the asymptomatic client may initially present solely with abnormal blood work on routine screening, whereas others may complain of dyspnea, fatigue, bounding pulses, palpitations, and a roaring pulsatile sound in the ears. As the anemia progresses, the client is at risk for lethargy, confusion, and other potentially life-threatening complications (Leung, 2019). Although there are a variety of types and etiologies of anemia, this section will focus on three that are most appropriate to manage in primary care: iron, vitamin B12, and folate deficiencies.

The major causes of iron deficiency are decreased dietary intake, reduced absorption, and blood loss (Auerbach, 2019). As blood loss is the most common etiology, the provider should inquire about a history of traumatic hemorrhage, hematemesis or melena, hemoptysis, menorrhagia, pregnancy/lactation/delivery, hematuria, frequent blood donation, excessive diagnostic blood testing, and gastrointestinal bleeding. Reduced iron absorption in conditions such as celiac disease or following bariatric surgery is an additional possible cause of iron deficiency (Auerbach, 2019). The cause of the deficiency must be identified and corrected by the primary care practitioner in collaboration with the specialty provider if indicated. The treatment of iron deficiency anemia depends on the severity of the condition. Once the course has been addressed, mild-to-moderate cases can be managed with oral supplementation, yet more severe anemia involves evaluation by a specialist and management via transfusion.

Fast Facts

Some special populations such as those with inflammatory bowel disease or chronic kidney disease may require intravenous iron supplementation (Auerbach, 2020).

Deficiencies of vitamin B12 can be anticipated in those who report a reduced intake of animal products or follow a strict vegan diet, in clients with decreased absorption (e.g., Crohn's disease, celiac disease, or pancreatic insufficiency), autoimmune disease (e.g., thyroid disease, vitiligo, pernicious anemia), or those on certain medications (e.g., metformin, histamine receptor antagonists, or proton pump inhibitors; Means & Fairfield, 2019a). Deficiency of folate is expected in those with a decreased intake of fresh vegetables and fortified grains or who consume alcohol in excess, in clients following gastric bypass surgery or are undergoing hemodialysis, and in those who use medication such as methotrexate or sulfasalazine (Means & Fairfield, 2019a). Once the source of the deficiency has been identified and addressed, the treatment of these deficiencies involves replacement that can be oral or parenteral depending on the severity of the condition. Typically, parenteral administration should be considered when the anemia is severe, the patient is symptomatic, or in cases of impaired absorption (Means & Fairfield, 2019b).

Thrombocytopenia

Thrombocytopenia is often discovered incidentally by the primary care provider while reviewing the results of routine diagnostic testing. The comprehensive history should include inquiry of easy bruising or petechiae, melena, rashes, fevers, and bleeding, and the physical examination should focus on signs of bleeding and evaluate for splenomegaly, hepatomegaly, lymphadenopathy, petechiae, purpura, bruising, and neurologic system changes. The etiology may not be obvious, so additional investigation is required, keeping in mind that a platelet count less than 5×10^3 per μL constitutes a hematologic emergency where prompt referral is indicated (Gauer & Braun, 2012). Various conditions can present with thrombocytopenia. Examples are described by Gauer and Braun (2012) and are provided in Box 8.2.

BOX 8.2 CONDITIONS THAT MAY PRESENT WITH THROMBOCYTOPENIA

Acute infection	Hematologic disorders
Heparin-induced thrombocytopenia	Preeclampsia
Liver disease	HELLP (hemolysis, elevated liver enzymes, and a low platelet count) syndrome
Thrombotic thrombocytopenic purpura	Gestational thrombocytopenia
Disseminated intravascular coagulation	Pseudothrombocytopenia
Hemolytic uremic syndrome	Drug-induced thrombocytopenia
Alcohol abuse	Nutritional deficiencies
Pulmonary emboli	Pulmonary hypertension

Source: Data from Gauer, R., & Braun, M. (2012). Thrombocytopenia. American Family Physician, 85(6), 612–622.

Treating the secondary cause of the thrombocytopenia most often results in a normalization of the platelet count. Consultation with a hematologist, however, should be considered in the event the client is hospitalized, with systemic disease, or if thrombocytopenia worsens or persists despite initial therapies (Gauer & Braun, 2012).

Leukocytosis

It is often the primary care provider who is faced with a client with an elevated white blood cell count. Although this diagnostic finding has many potential etiologies, including malignant and nonmalignant causes, and leukocytosis is a common sign of bacterial infection, this finding should prompt the provider to consider other conditions (Riley & Rupert, 2015). For example, Riley and Rupert (2015) report that stressors capable of causing an acute leukocytosis include surgery, exercise, trauma, and emotional stress, and other nonmalignant etiologies of leukocytosis include medications, asplenia, smoking, obesity, and chronic inflammatory conditions.

Symptoms that may suggest hematologic malignancy include fever, weight loss, bruising, or fatigue. Here, a referral to a hematologist/oncologist is indicated (Riley & Rupert, 2015). These authors go on to describe that the initial laboratory evaluation should include a repeat confirmatory complete blood count, as well as differential and peripheral blood smear. Depending on the client history and examination findings, the seasoned clinician will consider cultures of blood, urine, and joint or body fluid aspirates; rheumatologic studies; mononucleosis; serologic titers; and radiologic studies such as chest radiography, computed tomography, or bone scan.

MANAGEMENT OF PRIMARY CARE CONDITION IN THE ONCOLOGY PATIENT

Cancer patients and cancer survivors present to the primary care settings for the management of many of the same conditions discussed in other chapters. However, these clients may have some unique primary care needs. For example, while undergoing cancer treatment, clients may be at higher risk for infection. When no longer in active treatment, the literature suggests that these clients' needs include surveillance for recurrence, screening for the development of secondary cancers, monitoring and intervention for the long-term and late physical and psychological effects of cancer and its treatment (e.g., pain, fatigue, cardiotoxicity, neuropathy, hearing loss, infection, psychological distress, insomnia, infertility, sexual dysfunction), management of comorbid conditions, and routine preventive and primary care (Nekhlyudov & Snyder, 2019).

A healthy lifestyle that includes good nutritional habits, physical activity as tolerated, smoking cessation, limited alcohol intake, stress reduction, and management of comorbidities is to be promoted by the primary care provider in collaboration with the oncologist. Regular age-appropriate health maintenance activities should continue unless contraindicated.

The oncologist is to be consulted to discuss management planning in the event a new health condition develops. There may be a need for collaboration to take place between primary care, oncology, pharmacy, and other providers in cases where the client is undergoing treatment/maintenance/prevention therapies, and additional agents are being considered or added by multiple providers.

- A history of physical abuse must be considered and excluded in the client who presents with abnormal bruising or bleeding.
- As blood loss is the most common etiology of iron deficiency anemia, the provider should inquire about a history of traumatic hemorrhage, hematemesis or melena, hemoptysis, menorrhagia, pregnancy/lactation/delivery, hematuria, frequent blood donation, excessive diagnostic blood testing, and gastrointestinal bleeding.
- Deficiencies of vitamin B12 can be anticipated in clients who report a reduced intake of animal products or follow a strict vegan diet, in those with decreased absorption and autoimmune disease, or in those who are on certain medications.
- Deficiency of folate is expected in clients with decreased intake, in those following gastric bypass surgery or who are undergoing hemodialysis, and in those who are on certain medications.
- A platelet count $<5 \times 10^3$ per μL constitutes a hematologic emergency where prompt referral is indicated.
- Stressors capable of causing an acute leukocytosis include surgery, exercise, trauma, and emotional stress, and other nonmalignant etiologies of leukocytosis include medications, asplenia, smoking, obesity, and chronic inflammatory conditions.

(continued)

(continued)

- Surveillance for recurrence, screening for the development of secondary cancers, monitoring and intervention for the long-term and late physical and psychological effects of cancer and its treatment, management of comorbid conditions, and routine preventive care are important elements of primary care following cancer treatment.

SUMMARY

This journey through the subspecialties continued with a collaborative clinical practice session with physician specialists and nurse practitioners practicing in specialty settings. Clients presented with common complaints related to the hematologic–oncologic systems that often begin with their visit to the primary care provider. This clinical immersion experience led to the identification of conditions that the primary care provider is expected to diagnose or perhaps initiate management of, as well as those that are more appropriately managed in collaboration with a hematologist or oncologist. As always, effective management plans can only be developed once the provider has identified the correct etiology.

References

Auerbach, M. (2019). *Causes and diagnosis of iron deficiency and iron deficiency anemia in adults.* UpToDate. Retrieved from https://www.uptodate.com/contents/causes-and-diagnosis-of-iron-deficiency-and-iron-deficiency-anemia-in-adults

Auerbach, M. (2020). *Treatment of iron deficiency anemia in adults.* UpToDate. Retrieved from https://www.uptodate.com/contents/treatment-of-iron-deficiency-anemia-in-adults

Gauer, R., & Braun, M. (2012). Thrombocytopenia. *American Family Physician, 85*(6), 612–622.

Leung, L. (2019). *Approach to the adult with anemia.* UpToDate. Retrieved from https://www.uptodate.com/contents/approach-to-the-adult-with-anemia?search=anemia&source=search_result&selectedTitle=1~150&usage_type=default&display_rank=1

Means, R., & Fairfield, K. (2019a). *Clinical manifestations and diagnosis of vitamin B12 and folate deficiency.* UpToDate. Retrieved from https://www.uptodate.com/contents/clinical-manifestations-and-diagnosis-of-vitamin-b12-and-folate-deficiency

Means, R., & Fairfield, K. (2019b). *Treatment of vitamin B12 and folate deficiencies.* UpToDate. Retrieved from https://www.uptodate.com/contents/treatment-of-vitamin-b12-and-folate-deficiencies?search=vitamin%20 b12%20and%20folate%20deficiency&source=search_result&selectedTitl e=2~150&usage_type=default&display_rank=2

Nekhlyudov, L., & Snyder, C. (2019). *Overview of cancer survivorship care for primary care and oncology providers.* UpToDate. Retrieved from https:// www.uptodate.com/contents/overview-of-cancer-survivorship-care-for -primary-care-and-oncology-providers?search=cancer%20survivorship &source=search_result&selectedTitle=1~150&usage_type=default &display_rank=1

Neutze, D., & Roque, J. (2016). Clinical evaluation of bleeding and bruising in primary care. *American Family Physician, 93*(4), 279–286.

Riley, L., & Rupert, J. (2015). Evaluation of patients with leukocytosis. *American Family Physician, 92*(11), 1004–1011.

9

Practice Essentials for Infectious Disease

This journey through the subspecialties continues with some of the most common complaints that result in the client's visit to the primary care provider—infection. As always, effective management plans can only be developed once the provider has identified the correct source of the infection and corresponding pathology.

LYME DISEASE

In certain higher-risk regions of the country, clients commonly present to primary care settings with concern following a tick bite, or with symptoms that may, in fact, be related to Lyme disease. Evidence suggests that clients who are treated with the appropriate course of antibiotic therapy in the early stages of the disease often experience a complete and rapid recovery. In a small percentage of clients, fatigue and myalgias may persist for longer than 6 months and is referred to as posttreatment Lyme disease syndrome or more commonly chronic Lyme disease (Centers for Disease Control and Prevention [CDC], n.d.-f).

Current standards of care include initiation of oral antibiotic therapy that includes doxycycline (100 mg twice a day for 10–21 days), amoxicillin (500 mg three times a day for 14–21 days), or cefuroxime axetil (500 mg twice a day for 14–21 days). Clients with more severe illness affecting the neurological or cardiac forms of the condition may require penicillin or ceftriaxone intravenously. When the client is intolerant to the recommended therapies, macrolides such as azithromycin, clarithromycin, or erythromycin are acceptable, with lower efficacy (CDC, n.d.-f).

TRAVEL MEDICINE

As the number of international travelers continues to grow, so does the risk of exposure to communicable diseases. Primary care providers are frequently consulted on measures to avoid illness and remain healthy both during and following international travel. As always, the skillful practitioner is careful to conduct a comprehensive assessment of travel plans, which includes location of travel, dates of travel, duration of travel, accommodations, and planned activities (Kamata, Birrer, & Tokuda, 2017).

Potential risks should be presented and discussed. Examples include accidental injury (e.g., motor vehicle accidents, drowning, diving), environmental hazards (e.g., sunburn, jet lag), crime/assault, underlying medical/psychological conditions, dehydration, animal bites, insect stings, and altitude-related illness. The incidence of infectious disease is very high among travelers, yet causes only 1% of travel deaths. Some common infectious diseases that place international travelers at risk include malaria, tuberculosis, diarrhea, schistosomiasis, leishmaniasis, leptospirosis, rabies, poliomyelitis, dengue, yellow fever, meningococcal meningitis, measles, Ebola, or Japanese encephalitis (Kamata et al., 2017).

Age-related issues, underlying illness, immunosuppression, pregnancy, allergies, and vaccination status should be assessed. Conditions such as inflammatory bowel disease, congestive heart failure, or chronic obstructive pulmonary disease may pose higher risk due to lengthy and/or difficult travel and increased bouts of traveler's diarrhea. The client must understand the importance of fitness for travel, necessary precautions (e.g., food, water, insect repellent), medication management, risk of exposure to sexually transmitted infection, and access to/insurance coverage for international healthcare/hospitalization (Kamata et al., 2017).

Preventive care is an essential part of planning for international travel. The vaccines commonly indicated for international travel can be found in Box 9.1, and adequate timing must be allocated to complete the necessary vaccination schedule and allow for the traveling client to develop the appropriate immunity (Kamata et al., 2017):

BOX 9.1 COMMON VACCINES FOR INTERNATIONAL TRAVEL

Diphtheria	Meningococcus	Rubella
Hepatitis A	Mumps	Tetanus
Hepatitis B	Pertussis	Typhoid fever

(continued)

(continued)

Influenza	Pneumococcus	Varicella
Japanese encephalitis	Poliomyelitis	Yellow fever
Measles	Rabies	

Source: Data from Kamata, K., Birrer, R., & Tokuda, Y. (2017). Travel medicine: Part 1—The basics. *Journal of General and Family Medicine, 18*(2), 52–55. doi:10.1002/jgf2.39

The client should be instructed on the use of prophylaxis and self-care medications. These medications include antimalarials (e.g., chloroquine, atovaquone/proguanil, doxycycline, mefloquine, primaquine) and those used to treat diarrheal illness, high altitude (e.g., acetazolamide, dexamethasone), and motion sickness (e.g., scopolamine, dimenhydrinate), as well as a travel emergency kit (e.g., thermometer, medical records, over-the-counter and prescription medications, first aid supplies; Kamata et al., 2017). The CDC website offers a wealth of information for both the provider and the international traveler (CDC, n.d.-e).

METHICILLIN-RESISTANT *STAPHYLOCOCCUS AUREUS*

The client often presents to primary care settings complaining of a lesion, perhaps related to an insect bite. The site may be described as a furuncle, carbuncle, abscess, or boil, which is purulent in nature, with a palpable fluid-filled cavity, a yellow or white center, and a central point or "head." Often, it is draining pus, or pus can be aspirated with a needle or syringe. Methicillin-resistant *Staphylococcus aureus* (MRSA) should be considered in the differential diagnosis in this type of soft tissue infection (CDC, n.d.-c).

When MRSA is suspected, the skillful clinician drains the lesion, sends the drainage for culture and susceptibility testing, advises the client on wound care, and discusses a follow-up plan with the client—particularly, in the event they develop systemic symptoms or worsening of local symptoms, or if symptoms do not improve within 48 hours. Empiric outpatient options for antimicrobial treatment if MRSA is considered include clindamycin, tetracyclines (e.g., doxycycline or minocycline), or trimethoprim–sulfamethoxazole as MRSA is resistant to penicillin and cephalosporins and resistance is common in fluoroquinolones and macrolides. In the event systemic symptoms are present, or the client presents with severe local symptoms, has a history of immunosuppression, or fails to respond to incision and drainage, the provider should consider coverage with antimicrobial therapy for MRSA in addition to incision and drainage (CDC, n.d.-d).

ADULT IMMUNIZATION SCHEDULE

It is most often the primary care provider who advises the adult client on the importance of immunization adherence and relevant updates in the adult immunization schedule. For instance, for the 2018 to 2019 period, any influenza vaccine appropriate for the age and health status of the patient may be used, including live-attenuated influenza vaccines that previously were not recommended in the United States. Live-attenuated influenza vaccination is an option for the adult nonpregnant client up to the age of 49 years without immunocompromised or related conditions (e.g., HIV, anatomical or functional asplenia, cerebrospinal fluid leak, cochlear implant) or who is not a household contact of or caregiver to those who are severely immunocompromised.

Fast Facts

Adults with end-stage renal disease, heart or lung disease, chronic liver disease, or diabetes are precautioned against receiving live-attenuated influenza vaccination. In general, those with a history of Guillain–Barré syndrome within 6 weeks of a previous dose of influenza vaccine should not be vaccinated (CDC, n.d.-a, n.d.-b; Kim & Hunter, 2019).

Hepatitis B vaccine is recommended for adults; there are two- and three-dose alternatives available, and a vaccine from the same manufacturer should be used to complete the series when possible. Hepatitis A is indicated in certain populations such as homeless people, those with chronic liver disease or clotting factor disorders, at-risk international travelers, those with close contact to an international adoptee, men who have sex with men, those who use injection or noninjection drugs, those who work with hepatitis A virus in a laboratory or nonhuman primates infected with the virus, or any client who is not at risk but wants protection against the virus (Kim & Hunter, 2019).

Additional adult vaccinations to consider include meningitis B vaccine, human papillomavirus (HPV) vaccine, and recombinant zoster vaccine (RZV). The HPV vaccine is not recommended for pregnant clients, and pregnant women should delay RZV if indicated until after pregnancy. The zoster vaccine live is contraindicated in pregnancy (Kim & Hunter, 2019). Furthermore, tetanus, diphtheria, and acellular pertussis vaccines are recommended for every pregnancy. Pneumococcal vaccination coverage is recommended for the older adult clients (one to two doses depending on indication), and measles, mumps, and rubella and varicella vaccinations are also indicated for those adult clients without evidence of immunity (Kim & Hunter, 2019).

ANTIMICROBIAL STEWARDSHIP

It has been well documented that the overuse of antimicrobial agents fosters the spread of antimicrobial resistance, and despite this growing public health threat, inappropriate prescribing practices in primary care remain a common problem (Irwin et al., 2014). The risks of antibiotic overuse or overprescribing include not only increases in this antibiotic resistance but also may lead to increases in disease severity, disease length, health complications and adverse effects, risk of death, healthcare costs, rehospitalization, and a need for medical treatment of health problems that previously may have resolved on their own (Llor & Bjerrum, 2014).

Current evidence suggests that prescribers may practice habits such as prescribing for the wrong indication or using unnecessary broad-spectrum agents due to provider's knowledge gaps, practice demand, inability to distinguish between bacterial and viral infections, perceived patient perception, time necessary to explain why antibiotics are not indicated, and/or health beliefs of the provider (Irwin et al., 2014). It has, therefore, been concluded that multifaceted interventions that include a plan to provide active clinician education combined with clinician decision support systems appear to be the most effective in changing antibiotic-prescribing behaviors (Irwin et al., 2014). Electronic health records that prompt at the point of prescribing may be one solution to promote proper prescribing practices, and future inquiry in this area is needed. Some common conditions where antibiotics are often improperly prescribed are summarized by Irwin et al. (2014) and provided in Box 9.2.

CLOSTRIDIUM DIFFICILE

It has been reported that *Clostridium difficile* has emerged as the leading cause of nosocomial infectious diarrhea worldwide, and antibiotic use continues to be the predominant risk factor. It has been

BOX 9.2 CONDITIONS WHERE ANTIBIOTICS ARE COMMONLY PRESCRIBED IMPROPERLY

Nonspecific upper respiratory infection	Acute bronchitis
Acute rhinosinusitis	Pharyngitis
Acute otitis media	Urinary tract infection
Skin and soft tissue infection	Community-acquired pneumonia

Source: Irwin, A., Moore, S., Price, C., Jenkins, T., DeAlleaume, L., & West, D. (2014). Advances in the prevention and control of HAIs. *Agency for Healthcare Research and Quality*. Retrieved from ahrq.gov/hai/patient-safety-resources/advances-in-hai/hai-article6.html

further described that other factors that have contributed to this disease include age >65 years; host immunity; comorbid conditions such as irritable bowel disease, use of gastric acid–altering medications, antiperistaltic medications, or proton pump inhibitors (evidence is mixed); history of gastrointestinal surgery; peripartum females; hospitalization (particularly stays in the ICU) or stays in long-term care facilities; contact with spores on hands or objects; contaminated food, soil, water, or pets; and the use of chemotherapeutic agents, fluoroquinolone antibiotics, or clindamycin. Recent epidemic outbreaks have led to hypervirulent strains resulting in severe disease, disease reoccurrence, or even death (Bennett, 2012).

Efficient and effective diagnosis and management remain a challenge to the provider as treatment options are limited. The gold standard for diagnosis remains to be the cell culture cytotoxic assay. The key to containing this public health challenge includes preventing and controlling the disease through good antibiotic stewardship, proper hand hygiene, and conscientious environmental disinfection. As alcohol-based sanitizers have been proven ineffective in killing the spores, handwashing using soap and water must be encouraged. The first episode of mild-to-moderate disease should no longer be treated with metronidazole, as the latest standards recommend either vancomycin or fidaxomicin. The dosage is vancomycin 125 mg orally four times per day or fidaxomicin 200 mg twice daily for 10 days (Bennett, 2012; McDonald et al., 2018). A test-of-cure is not a standard of practice, and as always, more complicated cases or those unresponsive to standard therapies should involve consultation with a specialty provider.

Fast Facts

- The evidence suggests that clients who are treated with the appropriate course of antibiotic therapy in the early stages of Lyme disease often experience a complete and rapid recovery.
- The vaccines commonly indicated for international travel include diphtheria, hepatitis A, hepatitis B, tetanus, pertussis, typhoid fever, measles, rabies, mumps, meningococcus, rubella, poliomyelitis, varicella, Japanese encephalitis, pneumococcus, yellow fever, and influenza.
- Empiric outpatient options for antimicrobial treatment if MRSA is considered include clindamycin, tetracyclines (e.g., doxycycline or minocycline), or trimethoprim–sulfamethoxazole as MRSA is resistant to penicillin and cephalosporins and resistance is common in fluoroquinolones and macrolides.
- Adults with end-stage renal disease, heart or lung disease, chronic liver disease, or diabetes are precautioned against receiving live-attenuated influenza vaccination.
- The risks of antibiotic overuse or overprescribing include not only increases in this antibiotic resistance but also may lead to increases in disease severity, disease length, health complications and adverse effects, risk of death, healthcare costs, rehospitalization, and a need for medical treatment of health problems that previously may have resolved on their own.
- Factors that have contributed to *Clostridium difficile* include age >65 years, host immunity, comorbid conditions such as irritable bowel disease, use of gastric acid–altering medications, antiperistaltic medications, or proton pump inhibitors (evidence is mixed); history of gastrointestinal surgery; peripartum females; hospitalization (particularly stays in the ICU) or stays in long-term care facilities; contact with spores on hands or objects; contaminated food, soil, water, or pets; and the use of chemotherapeutic agents, fluoroquinolone antibiotics, or clindamycin.

SUMMARY

This journey through the subspecialties continued with a variety of collaborative clinical practice sessions with physician specialists and nurse practitioners practicing in specialty settings. Clients presented with common complaints of infection that often begin with their visit to the primary care provider. This clinical immersion experience led to the identification of hot topics that the primary/urgent care nurse practitioner is expected to diagnose or perhaps initiate management of. As always, effective management plans can only be developed once the provider has identified the correct etiology.

References

Bennett, J. (2012). *Clostridium difficile*: A new look at an old but increasingly deadly infection. *JAAPA, 25*(1), 32–36. doi:10.1097/01720610-201201000-00007

Centers for Disease Control and Prevention. (n.d.-a). *ACIP vaccine recommendations and guidelines.* Retrieved from www.cdc.gov/vaccines/hcp/acip-recs/index.html

Centers for Disease Control and Prevention. (n.d.-b). *Immunization schedules.* Retrieved from www.cdc.gov/vaccines/schedules

Centers for Disease Control and Prevention. (n.d.-c). *Methicillin-resistant* Staphylococcus aureus *(MRSA): Outpatient management.* Retrieved from https://www.cdc.gov/mrsa/healthcare/outpatient.html

Centers for Disease Control and Prevention. (n.d.-d). *Outpatient management of skin and soft tissue infections in the era of community-associated MRSA.* Retrieved from https://www.cdc.gov/mrsa/pdf/flowchart_pstr.pdf

Centers for Disease Control and Prevention. (n.d.-e). *Travelers' health.* Retrieved from www.cdc.gov/travel

Centers for Disease Control and Prevention. (n.d.-f). *Treatment.* Retrieved from https://www.cdc.gov/lyme/treatment/index.html

Irwin, A., Moore, S., Price, C., Jenkins, T., DeAlleaume, L., & West, D. (2014). Advances in the prevention and control of HAIs. *Agency for Healthcare Research and Quality.* Retrieved from ahrq.gov/hai/patient-safety-resources/advances-in-hai/hai-article6.html

Kamata, K., Birrer, R., & Tokuda, Y. (2017). Travel medicine: Part 1-The basics. *Journal of General and Family Medicine, 18*(2), 52–55. doi:10.1002/jgf2.39

Kim, D., & Hunter, P. (2019). Recommended adult immunization schedule, United States, 2019. *Annals of Internal Medicine.* Retrieved from https://annals.org/aim/fullarticle/2723806/recommended-adult-immunization-schedule-united-states-2019?_ga=2.96582815.1631277570.1575313238-118521563.1575313238

Llor, C., & Bjerrum, L. (2014). Antimicrobial resistance: Risk associated with antibiotic overuse and initiatives to reduce the problem. *Therapeutic Advances in Drug Safety, 5*(6), 229–241. doi:10.1177/2042098614554919

McDonald, L. C., Gerding, D. N., Johnson, S., Bakken, J. S., Carroll, K. C., Coffin, S. E., & Wilcox, M. H. (2018). Clinical Practice Guidelines for *Clostridium difficile* infection in adults and children: 2017 update by the Infectious Diseases Society of America (IDSA) and Society for Healthcare Epidemiology of America (SHEA). *Clinical Infectious Diseases, 66*(7), e1–e48. doi:10.1093/cid/cix1085

10

Practice Essentials for Nephrology

The adult client may present to the primary care setting with a variety of symptoms related to the kidney. Although many of these are appropriate for the primary care provider to diagnose and manage, some conditions may be persistent or significant enough to be referred to the nephrologist. As there is some overlap with the urological system, a number of conditions related to the kidney such as pyelonephritis, nephrolithiasis, and renal cysts are presented in Chapter 20, Practice Essentials for Urology. The skillful provider is knowledgeable on the standards of care for the client with a nephrological condition as well as the red flags to assess and refer for a consultation with the correct specialty provider.

CHRONIC KIDNEY DISEASE

Evidence suggests that the early identification and timely referral of the client with chronic kidney disease (CKD) to a nephrologist for management has demonstrated improved healthcare outcomes and that a team approach to care that includes the primary care provider, nephrologist, and other specialists such as nephrology nurses, social workers, nutritionists, and renal education specialists is critical to preserve and maintain renal function and avoid the need for dialysis or transplant (Khanna, 2011). The seasoned primary care provider is knowledgeable that the estimated glomerular filtration rate (GFR) is the best test to measure kidney function and determine kidney disease stage and is calculated based on serum creatinine, age, race, and gender, as well as on the current standards to stage CKD, which are presented in Table 10.1.

Table 10.1

Stages of CKD			
Stage 1	Normal or high GFR	GFR > 90 mL/min	90%–100% kidney function
Stage 2	Mild CKD	GFR = 60–89 mL/min	89%–60% kidney function
Stage 3A	Moderate CKD	GFR = 45–59 mL/min	45%–59% kidney function
Stage 3B	Moderate CKD	GFR = 30–44 mL/min	30%–44% kidney function
Stage 4	Severe CKD	GFR = 15–29 mL/min	15%–29% kidney function
Stage 5	End-stage CKD	GFR < 15 mL/min	<15% kidney function

CKD, chronic kidney disease; GFR, glomerular filtration rate.
Source: Data from National Kidney Foundation. (2018). *Estimated glomerular filtration rate (eGFR)*. Retrieved from https://www.kidney.org/atoz/content/gfr

The initial workup of the client at risk for chronic renal disease would also consist of urinalysis for proteinuria and/or hematuria, as well as a renal ultrasound, while a nephrology consult and evaluation for renal biopsy are other important elements of the initial management plan for impaired renal function (Rosenberg, 2019). Rosenberg (2019) goes on to describe how the gradual decline in renal function is initially asymptomatic; however, with advancing renal failure, clients may present with manifestations of hyperkalemia, metabolic acidosis, hypertension, anemia, and/or mineral and bone disorders. Furthermore, the signs and symptoms of CKD to observe for include nausea, vomiting, loss of appetite, fatigue and weakness, sleep problems, changes in urinary patterns, decreased mental sharpness, muscle twitches and cramps, lower extremity edema, pruritus, chest pain, dyspnea, and/or hypertension that is difficult to control. Therefore, the skillful primary care practitioner is careful to observe and monitor at-risk clients such as those with diabetes, high blood pressure, and cardiovascular disease; who are smokers, obese, African American, Native American, or Asian American; and those with a family history of kidney disease, abnormal kidney structure, or advancing age and refer accordingly (Mayo Clinic, 2019). Additionally, the primary care provider must be competent in identifying and avoiding recommending drugs/drug classes that may impact renal function such as aminoglycoside antibiotics, nonsteroidal anti-inflammatory drugs, and radiographic contrast when managing the primary care needs of the client with CKD, as well as to promote the control of comorbid conditions that may have an impact on renal function such as hypertension, hyperlipidemia, and diabetes and to support the client in protein restriction and smoking cessation (Rosenberg, 2019). Management of blood pressure, lipids, and blood glucose in clients with impaired renal function is described in the cardiology and endocrine chapters (Chapter 4, Practice Essentials for Cardiology, and Chapter 6, Practice Essentials for Endocrinology).

Fast Facts

The primary care provider may also play a role in supporting the client with CKD who presents with other factors related to their impaired renal function. Examples include sexual dysfunction, thyroid dysfunction, increased risk for infection, and altered guidelines for immunization. For instance, the KDIGO 2012 Clinical Practice Guideline for the Evaluation and Management of Chronic Kidney Disease (2013) includes the following immunization recommendations for the adult client:

- Offer adults with all stages of CKD annual influenza vaccination unless contraindicated.
- Offer adults with stages 4 and 5 CKD who are at high risk of progression of CKD immunization against hepatitis B and confirm response by immunologic testing.
- Offer adults with stages 4 and 5 CKD polyvalent pneumococcal vaccination unless contraindicated and offer revaccination within 5 years.

Finally, as there will likely be an increased risk for retinopathy, cataracts, or glaucoma, regular referrals for screening by an ophthalmologist are an additional important component of the primary care management of a client with chronic renal disease (Bodaghi, Massamba, & Izzedine, 2014). Other specialists such as cardiologists and/or endocrinologists may play a key role in the management of conditions such as hypertension, hyperlipidemia, and diabetes in the client with CKD.

GLOMERULONEPHRITIS

The primary care provider often encounters abnormalities on urinalysis in the symptomatic or asymptomatic client. Glomerulonephritis should be considered when a routine urinalysis is abnormal demonstrating red blood cells and red cell casts, white blood cells, and increased protein. Increased levels of serum creatinine or urea are additional indicators of glomerulonephritis (Mayo Clinic, 2020). Renal ultrasound and/or CT scan may be indicated in these clients.

As a renal biopsy is almost always necessary to confirm a diagnosis of glomerulonephritis, timely referral to a nephrologist is indicated when the primary care provider is suspicious of glomerulonephritis. It has been reported that some cases of acute glomerulonephritis, especially those that follow a strep infection, may resolve without intervention; however, if there is an underlying cause, such as hypertension, infection, or autoimmune disease, management of the glomerulonephritis will be directed to the underlying cause with the goal of treatment as renal protection from further damage (Mayo Clinic, 2020).

NEPHROTIC SYNDROME

The adult client who presents to the primary care setting with edema, fatigue, heavy proteinuria, hypoalbuminemia, and hyperlipidemia without evidence of heart failure or liver disease should be evaluated for nephrotic syndrome. Underlying conditions such as type 2 diabetes mellitus and systemic lupus erythematosus can cause nephrotic syndrome, as can some secondary causes such as metabolic or neoplastic disease, amyloidosis, immunologic conditions, erythema multiforme, Sjögren syndrome, cancers (e.g., lung, breast, colon, stomach, kidney, leukemia, lymphoma, melanoma, multiple myeloma), medication/drug use (e.g., heroin, lithium, nonsteroidal anti-inflammatory drugs), endocarditis, syphilis, malaria, Epstein–Barr virus, hepatitis B or C, herpes zoster, HIV, insect stings, poison ivy or oak, malignant hypertension, preeclampsia, or sarcoidosis (Kodner, 2016).

New-onset edema of the lower extremities is the most common presenting symptom of nephrotic syndrome. The edema may extend to the lower abdomen or genitalia depending on disease severity. Kodner (2016) describes ascites, periorbital edema, hypertension, foamy urine, dyspnea on exertion, weight gain, and pleural effusion as other possible features the client may present with. Often, a renal biopsy is indicated for diagnosis. Therefore, a nephrologist should be consulted for diagnosis and management due to the risk of the major complications of this condition such as venous thrombosis, infection, hyperlipidemia, or renal failure (Kodner, 2016). In general, management will involve sodium restriction and management of edema with diuretic therapies. Other interventions may include anticoagulation, the treatment and prevention of infection, the management of dyslipidemia, and immunosuppressive therapies (Kodner, 2016).

Fast Facts

- The estimated GFR is the best test to measure kidney function and determine kidney disease stage.
- The signs and symptoms of CKD include nausea, vomiting, loss of appetite, fatigue and weakness, sleep problems, changes in urinary patterns, decreased mental sharpness, muscle twitches and cramps, lower extremity edema, pruritus, chest pain, dyspnea, and/or hypertension that is difficult to control.
- Glomerulonephritis should be considered when a routine urinalysis is abnormal demonstrating red blood cells and red cell casts, white blood cells, and increased protein, and there is indication of increased serum creatinine or urea.
- New-onset edema of the lower extremities is the most common presenting symptom of nephrotic syndrome, and when the edema extends to the lower abdomen or genitalia, there may be an indication of increased disease severity.

SUMMARY

This journey through the subspecialties continued with a collaborative clinical practice session with physician specialists and nurse practitioners practicing in specialty settings. Clients presented with common complaints related to the kidney that often begin with their visit to the primary care provider. This clinical immersion experience led to the identification of conditions that the primary care provider is expected to diagnose or perhaps initiate during the management of clients with a variety of conditions affecting the kidney. As always, effective management plans can only be developed once the provider has identified the correct etiology.

References

Bodaghi, B., Massamba, N., & Izzedine, H. (2014). The eye: A window on kidney diseases. *Clinical Kidney Journal, 7*(4), 337–338. doi:10.1093/ckj/sfu073

KDIGO. (2013). KDIGO 2012 clinical practice guideline for the evaluation and management of chronic kidney disease. *Kidney International Supplements, 3*, 5.

Khanna, R. (2011). Nephrology for primary care physicians. *Missouri Medicine, 108*(1), 23–24.

Kodner, C. (2016). Diagnosis and management of nephrotic syndrome in adults. *American Family Physician, 93*(6), 479–485.

Mayo Clinic. (2019). *Chronic kidney disease: Overview.* Retrieved from https://www.mayoclinic.org/diseases-conditions/chronic-kidney-disease/symptoms-causes/syc-20354521

Mayo Clinic. (2020). *Glomerulonephritis.* Retrieved from https://www.mayoclinic.org/diseases-conditions/glomerulonephritis/diagnosis-treatment/drc-20355710

National Kidney Foundation. (2018). *Estimated glomerular filtration rate (eGFR).* Retrieved from https://www.kidney.org/atoz/content/gfr

Rosenberg, M. (2019). *Overview of the management of chronic kidney disease in adults.* UpToDate. Retrieved from https://www.uptodate.com/contents/overview-of-the-management-of-chronic-kidney-disease-in-adults

11

Practice Essentials for Neurology

Clients often seek care in primary care settings for symptoms related to the neurologic system. At times, this is appropriate, and a diagnosis can be made and symptoms managed with optimal outcomes achieved. More severe, persistent, or difficult-to-control conditions may often require imaging studies to formulate a diagnosis/management plan and likely must be referred to a specialist or emergency services when indicated.

FATIGUE

Fatigue is a general complaint that can range from minimal and intermittent in nature to a chronic state that can result in tremendous cost and severely impact one's quality of life. Acute fatigue lasts <1 month, subacute 1–6 months, and chronic fatigue >6 months (Fosnocht & Ende, 2019). Symptoms are reported more commonly in female clients, and etiologies may range from various medical disorders to psychological conditions. Some possible causes of acute and chronic fatigue are summarized in Table 11.1 (Fosnocht & Ende, 2019).

The skillful practitioner is thoughtful in conducting a thorough health history (i.e., onset, course, duration, patterns, related factors, and impact) and a comprehensive physical examination—emphasizing general health status, thyroid examination, assessment for lymphadenopathy/hepatosplenomegaly, and evaluation of the cardiopulmonary and neuromuscular systems. Initial laboratory testing includes complete blood count, serum chemistries, thyroid-stimulating hormone, and creatine kinase if muscle pain/weakness

Table 11.1

Causes of Acute and Chronic Fatigue

Causes of Acute Fatigue	Causes of Subacute/Chronic Fatigue
Acute illness	Cardiopulmonary conditions: ■ Congestive heart failure, chronic obstructive pulmonary disease, sleep apnea
Fever	Endocrine/metabolic conditions: ■ Hypothyroidism, hyperthyroidism, chronic renal disease, chronic hepatic disease, adrenal insufficiency, electrolyte abnormalities
Influenza	Hematologic/neoplastic conditions: ■ Anemia, occult malignancy
Recent life stressor	Infectious diseases: ■ Mononucleosis syndrome, viral hepatitis, HIV infection, subacute bacterial endocarditis, tuberculosis
Recognizable medical condition	Rheumatologic conditions: ■ Fibromyalgia, polymyalgia rheumatica, systemic lupus erythematosus, rheumatoid arthritis, Sjögren's syndrome
Recognizable psychological condition	Psychological conditions: ■ Depression, anxiety disorder, somatization disorder
Recent increased intake of alcohol	Neurological conditions: ■ Multiple sclerosis
	Medication toxicity: ■ Benzodiazepines, antidepressants, muscle relaxants, antihistamines, β-blockers, opioids
	Substance use/abuse: ■ Alcohol, marijuana, opioids, cocaine, or other stimulants

Source: Data from Fosnocht, K., & Ende, J. (2019). *Approach to the adult patient with fatigue.* UpToDate. Retrieved from https://www.uptodate.com/contents/approach-to-the-adult-patient-with-fatigue/print

is present (Fosnocht & Ende, 2019). Furthermore, Fosnocht and Ende (2019) also recommend including appropriate cancer screening interventions based upon the client's age and sex to exclude common occult malignancies as a potential cause for fatigue. Any additional necessary workup is determined based on health history and related symptomatology.

The management of fatigue begins with the establishment of a supportive provider–client relationship. Underlying medical conditions are to be managed according to standards of care. Antidepressant therapy may be indicated (selective serotonin reuptake inhibitor or a serotonin-norepinephrine reuptake inhibitor), yet the empirical use of stimulants is not suggested. Cognitive behavioral therapy (CBT) and/or exercise therapy are recommended as tolerated (Fosnocht & Ende, 2019).

MUSCLE WEAKNESS

The client may present to primary care settings with a complaint of weakness. The symptoms of true muscle weakness must be differentiated from that of fatigue, as clients who complain of weakness may not be objectively weak when muscle strength is tested. A careful history and physical examination will permit the distinction between fatigue, motor impairment due to pain or joint dysfunction, and true weakness.

Fast Facts

The integral components of the health history of the client complaining of muscle weakness are as follows:

- Cardiopulmonary disease where the patient is limited by shortness of breath or chest pain
- Joint disease or joint pain
- Anemia
- Cachexia from malignancy or chronic infectious or inflammatory disease
- Depression
- Poor exercise tolerance (e.g., cannot climb stairs or comb hair due to heaviness or stiffness of limbs)
- Paresthesias
- Spasticity
- Medication, alcohol, or substance abuse

Source: Data from Miller, M. (2019). *Approach to the patient with muscle weakness*. Retrieved from https://www.uptodate.com/contents/muscle-examination-in-the-evaluation-of-weakness

Miller (2019) goes on to describe that true muscle weakness is assessed as symmetric or asymmetric and documented by formal muscle testing based upon a scale of 0 to 5 (Box 11.1).

BOX 11.1 MUSCLE TESTING SCALE

- 0—No muscle contraction
- 1—Flicker or trace of muscle contraction
- 2—Limb or joint movement possible only with gravity eliminated
- 3—Limb or joint movement against gravity only
- 4—Power decreased but limb or joint movement possible against resistance
- 5—Normal power against resistance

Source: Data from Miller, M. (2019). *Approach to the patient with muscle weakness*. UpToDate. Retrieved from https://www.uptodate.com/contents/muscle-examination-in-the-evaluation-of-weakness

Imaging studies, cerebrospinal fluid examination, and/or muscle biopsy may be necessary to identify the etiology of the symptoms. Depending upon the suspected site of the lesion, MRI of the brain and/or spinal cord, plain radiographs of the spine, radionuclide bone scanning, or CT scanning may be appropriate imaging modalities (Miller, 2019). At this time, the scope and breadth of the management plan may supersede the primary care setting, and consultation with a specialty provider may be appropriate. Patients who present with muscle weakness should also be assessed for respiratory muscle weakness, particularly in the presence of signs or symptoms of tachypnea, shortness of breath, or somnolence or a history of impaired swallowing, dysphonia, or nasal regurgitation (Miller, 2019). To extend the initial workup, the skillful practitioner may also include the following laboratory studies: chemistry and urinalysis which, when positive for blood in the urine, is suggestive of myoglobinuria; creatine kinase, aldolase, lactate dehydrogenase, and the aminotransferases which, when elevated, are highly suggestive of muscle diseases; and serologic tests including antinuclear antibodies, anti-Sjogren's-syndrome-related antigen A, anti-Sjogren's-syndrome-related antigen B, anti-Smith antibody, and anti-ribonucleoprotein, and antihistidyl-t-RNA synthase; antineutrophil cytoplasmic antibody titers, hepatitis B and C serologies, and cryoglobulins (Miller, 2019).

INSOMNIA

Clients will often present to primary care settings complaining of acute insomnia (<3 months) or chronic insomnia (inability to fall asleep, maintain sleep, or waking up early in the morning and not being able to return to sleep for at least three nights per week for 3 months or longer). Chronic insomnia can be problematic and affect functional health and quality of life, warranting further assessment (Cadet et al., 2019).

Fast Facts

Predisposing factors for chronic insomnia include female gender, age >60 years, inactive lifestyle, night-shift work, relationship problems, noise/light, traveling across time zones, and caring for a newborn, as well as other conditions such as stress, anxiety, depression, restless leg syndrome, chronic pain, asthma, chronic obstructive pulmonary disease, obstructive sleep apnea, head trauma, thyroid disorders, menopause symptoms, heartburn, irritable bowel syndrome, alcohol/caffeine use, pregnancy, and use of the following medications: psychostimulants and amphetamines, antiepileptic drugs, corticosteroids, cold medications, and decongestants (Cadet et al., 2019).

The seasoned provider is careful to conduct a thorough health history (including review of sleep logs and self-report instruments) and comprehensive physical examination in order to formulate the correct diagnosis and implement the proper management plan. Often, sleep studies are indicated to determine the diagnosis of insomnia. Once a diagnosis is made and any comorbidities are addressed, the initial management of insomnia involves nonpharmacologic modalities such as CBT as a first-line therapy; sleep hygiene education; sleep restriction (e.g., limiting naps to 30 minutes); stimulus control; exercise; avoidance of alcohol, caffeine, and certain foods (e.g., heavy or rich foods, fatty or fried meals, spicy dishes, citrus fruits, and carbonated drinks); and relaxation training. Pharmacologic interventions, such as melatonin receptor agonists, nonbenzodiazepine hypnotics, orexin receptor antagonists, antidepressants, benzodiazepines, or, although not Food and Drug Administration (FDA) regulated, herbs and supplements, such as melatonin, valerian root, kava, St. John's wort, lavender, and passionflower, may also be considered (Cadet et al., 2019).

HEADACHE

Headaches are a common complaint resulting in a visit to the primary care setting. A headache can result from a variety of conditions. Types include migraine, tension, or cluster headaches. More severe headaches can impair function, require bed rest, and lead to absence from work or school, and a diagnosis of migraines should be considered when the client presents with recurrent sinus headaches (Becker et al., 2015).

Imaging studies are not recommended for the routine assessment of the client with a headache. The skilled practitioner is cognizant of the key elements of a thorough history and comprehensive physical examination. As migraines are the most common type of headache, once a diagnosis is made, management involves preventative therapies such as lifestyle changes and the avoidance of triggers. Over-the-counter management of tension, cluster-type, and medication-overuse headaches is often ineffective, so the appropriate assessment and pharmacologic/nonpharmacologic management plan are critical (Becker et al., 2015).

As always, the seasoned provider is careful to assess for any red flags requiring emergent referral and care. These include thunderclap onset, fever, meningismus, papilledema with focal signs or reduced level of consciousness, and acute glaucoma. Other symptoms to be addressed urgently are as follows: temporal arteritis, relevant systemic illness, and elderly patients with a new headache involving cognitive change. Signs to investigate further include headache >3 days per month, cases where acute administration of medications is not effective, or disability despite acute administration of medication. Other types of headaches that should involve a referral to a specialist include hemicrania continua, new daily persistent headache, unexplained focal signs, atypical headaches, unusual headache precipitants, unusual aura symptoms, and onset after the age of 50 years (Becker et al., 2015).

Fast Facts

The behavioral management of headaches begins with keeping a headache diary (i.e., frequency, intensity, triggers, and medication). Then, lifestyle factors can be adjusted accordingly such as reducing caffeine, incorporating regular exercise, and avoiding irregular or inadequate sleep or meals. Often, the development and use of stress management strategies such as relaxation training, CBT, pacing activity, and/or biofeedback can be advised to manage headaches (Becker et al., 2015).

Becker et al. (2015) describe the first-line management of migraines, which includes ibuprofen 400 mg, aspirin 1,000 mg, naproxen sodium 500 to 550 mg, or acetaminophen 1,000 mg, and the second-line management of migraines, which involves oral, subcutaneous, or nasal triptans. The difficult-to-manage migraine headache can be treated with naproxen sodium in combination with a triptan. The first-line prophylactic treatment options are propranolol 20 mg BID, metoprolol 50 mg BID, nadolol 40 mg QD, amitriptyline 10 mg Q HS, or nortriptyline 10 mg Q HS, whereas second-line agents include topiramate 25 mg QD, candesartan 8 mg QD, or gabapentin 300 mg QD (Becker et al., 2015).

Tension headaches can be initially managed with ibuprofen 400 mg, aspirin 1,000 mg, naproxen sodium 500 to 550 mg, or acetaminophen 1,000 mg. First-line prophylactic management includes amitriptyline 10 to 100 mg QD or nortriptyline 10 to 100 mg QD, and second-line management includes mirtazapine 30 mg QD or venlafaxine 150 mg QD (Becker et al., 2015). Although an early specialist referral should be considered for cluster headaches, pharmacologic management may involve subcutaneous sumatriptan, intranasal zolmitriptan, and 100% oxygen, and first-line prophylactic treatment includes verapamil (Becker et al., 2015).

Overall, the optimal management of the primary care client initiates with the correct diagnosis and the understanding of limitations and need to consult with a specialty provider or refer for emergency management. Furthermore, as always, it is critical to assess for any comorbid conditions, which may limit or affect successful pharmacologic interventions. It is also crucial to educate the client on lifestyle factors, which may be headache triggers or interfering with a successful treatment plan.

DIZZINESS

Clients often present to primary care settings complaining of dizziness. A careful history on the timing (e.g., onset, duration, and evolution of dizziness) and triggers (e.g., actions, movements, trauma, or situations) and a comprehensive physical examination (including a cardiac and neurologic assessment, with attention to the head, eye, ear, nose, and throat, orthostatic blood pressure measurement, as dizziness from orthostatic hypotension occurs with movement to the upright position, nystagmus assessment, and the Dix–Hallpike maneuver for triggered vertigo) will promote the provider's ability to distinguish between vertigo, presyncope, disequilibrium, and lightheadedness. As many of these conditions may be nonspecific, this section will focus on dizziness and vertigo. Some common peripheral causes of dizziness and vertigo include benign paroxysmal positional vertigo, vestibular neuritis, Meniere disease, and otosclerosis, whereas possible central causes include vestibular migraine, cerebrovascular disease, or meningiomas. Other causes may be psychiatric in nature, medication-induced, orthostatic, or related to cardiovascular and/or metabolic conditions. In fact, vertigo can be a presenting symptom of an impending cerebrovascular event (Muncie, Sirmans, & James, 2017).

Although most patients presenting with dizziness do not require laboratory testing, clients with chronic medical conditions such as diabetes mellitus or hypertension may require blood glucose and electrolyte measurements and those with symptoms of cardiac disease should undergo electrocardiography, Holter monitoring, and carotid Doppler testing. Also, routine imaging is not indicated in the evaluation of the client with dizziness; in the event of any abnormal neurologic finding, including asymmetric or unilateral hearing loss, CT or MRI is recommended (Muncie et al., 2017).

When the client describes a sensation of self-motion when they are not moving or a sensation of distorted self-motion during normal head movement, they may, in fact, have vertigo. If the vertigo is triggered by a sudden change in position, such as a quick turn of the head or tipping head back in the shower, the provider may suspect benign paroxysmal positional vertigo. If a sensation of vertigo is described, the client should also be screened for hearing loss, which may suggest Meniere disease (Muncie et al., 2017).

Medications may result in dizziness in the older adult client. The evidence suggests that the use of five or more medications is associated with an increased risk of dizziness and that the older client is more susceptible.

Fast Facts

Examples of medications that can commonly cause dizziness in the adult client are as follows:

- Alcohol
- Antiepileptics
- Anti-infectives, such as quinolones
- Antiparkinsonian agents
- Glycosides
- Nitrates
- Sodium–glucose cotransporter-2 inhibitors
- Antiepileptics
- Antidiabetic agents
- Antirheumatic agents
- Antiarrhythmics
- Antihistamines

(continued)

(continued)

- Anti-influenza agents
- Attention deficit hyperactivity disorder agents
- Dipyridamole
- Phosphodiesterase type 5 inhibitors
- Urinary anticholinergics
- Benzodiazepines
- β-Adrenergic blockers
- Anticoagulants
- Antidementia agents
- Antihypertensives
- Antifungals
- Digitalis
- Narcotics
- Skeletal muscle relaxants
- Urinary and gastrointestinal antispasmodics
- Lithium
- Aminoglycosides
- Antithyroid agents

Source: Data from Muncie, H., Sirmans, S., & James, E. (2017). Dizziness: Approach to evaluation and management. *American Family Physician, 95*(3), 154–162.

As always, an effective management plan can be implemented once the correct diagnosis is made. For instance, pharmacologic agents are ineffective in the treatment of benign paroxysmal positional vertigo. Here, treatment consists of referral for a canalith repositioning procedure such as the Epley maneuver. If there is no improvement with repeated repositioning maneuvers, or if atypical or ongoing nystagmus with nausea is present, another cause of the symptoms should be considered (Muncie et al., 2017).

Vestibular neuritis, another common cause of vertigo, is thought to be viral in origin and is treated with antiemetic or antinausea medications for no more than 3 days. A referral for vestibular rehabilitation may also be effective. The symptoms of vertigo and associated nausea or vomiting can also be treated with a combination of antihistamine, antiemetic, or benzodiazepines. Systemic corticosteroids and antiviral medications have been found to be ineffective in the management of vestibular neuritis (Muncie et al., 2017).

Meniere disease causes severe enough vertigo to necessitate bed rest, nausea, vomiting, loss of balance, sudden slips or falls, headache, and unilateral hearing loss. It has been reported that these clients will manifest a unidirectional, horizontal–torsional nystagmus during the vertigo episodes. The first-line treatment involves lifestyle changes, including limiting dietary salt intake to <2,000 mg per day, reducing caffeine intake, and limiting alcohol to one drink per day, and thiazide diuretic therapy can be added daily if the symptoms are not controlled with these lifestyle changes (Muncie et al., 2017).

DEMENTIA

The adult or older adult client may present to the primary care setting reporting symptoms related to dementia. As this disease and its progression may be quite difficult for even the skilled practitioner to manage, it is likely best to refer the client to consult with specialty providers with expertise in this area such as neurology and/or a geriatrician. There are a number of well-documented reasons for referral. These include functional and memory decline, medication review, assessment of behavioral disturbances, and concerns about decision-making ability and client safety. Time constraints, inadequate knowledge, limited skill set, fear of making the accurate diagnosis, lack of remuneration, and lack of coordination between services further complicate the effective management of dementia and missed diagnosis of early dementia in primary care settings (Parmar et al., 2014). However, as always, it is critical that the primary care provider, who is the expert in the client's health history and overall health status, remain current on the standards of care and play an active role in the team approach to the management of the client with dementia, as well as to provide support to and educate family/caregivers on best practices and resources available to them to minimize caregiver stress and burden.

Parmar et al. (2014) report that high-quality dementia care involves a documented diagnosis of the dementia and its severity; cognitive testing such as the Mini-Mental State Examination; inquiry into basic activities of daily living; laboratory testing such as complete blood count and measurement of electrolytes, thyroid-stimulating hormone, and blood glucose, and calcium levels; and the identification of behavioral and psychological issues, caregiver burden, and safety issues such as wandering and driving. Guidance toward care in the community, the need for long-term care, the establishment of personal directives, power of attorney, and capacity assessment may also be indicated. Other concerns such as neglect and/or elder abuse should involve other multidisciplinary experts such as social workers. As longevity increases and the baby boomers continue to age and the rates of dementia continue to increase, evidence suggests a need to transition from fragmented models of dementia care to a more integrated approach to management that is more collaborative and consistent in the provision of services and avoids duplication. It very well may be the seasoned primary care practitioner who is charged to lead these efforts, and future inquiry into these types of models is encouraged (Parmar et al., 2014).

Fast Facts

- The management of fatigue begins with the establishment of a supportive provider–client relationship.
- Patients who present with muscle weakness should be assessed for respiratory muscle weakness, particularly in the presence of signs or symptoms of tachypnea, shortness of breath, or somnolence or a history of impaired swallowing, dysphonia, or nasal regurgitation, and referred appropriately.
- Pharmacologic interventions for insomnia, such as melatonin receptor agonists, nonbenzodiazepine hypnotics, orexin receptor antagonists, antidepressants, benzodiazepines, or, although not FDA regulated, herbs and supplements such as melatonin, valerian root, kava, St. John's wort, lavender, and passionflower may also be considered.
- Imaging studies are not recommended for the routine assessment of the client with a headache.
- The use of five or more medications is associated with an increased risk of dizziness, and the older client is more susceptible.
- As longevity increases and baby boomers continue to age and rates of dementia continue to increase, the evidence suggests a need to transition from fragmented models of dementia care to a more integrated approach to management that is more collaborative and consistent in the provision of services and avoids duplication.

SUMMARY

This journey through the subspecialties continued with a collaborative clinical practice session with physician specialists and nurse practitioners practicing in specialty settings. Clients presented with common neurological complaints that often begin with their visit to the primary care provider. This clinical immersion experience led to the identification of conditions that the primary care provider is expected to diagnose or perhaps initiate during the management of clients with a variety of conditions affecting the neurological system. As always, effective management plans can only be developed once the provider has identified the correct etiology.

References

Becker, W., Findlay, T., Moga, C., Scott, N., Harstall, C., & Taenzer, P. (2015). Guideline for primary care management of headache in adults. *Canadian Family Physician, 61*, 670–679.

Cadet, M., Tucker, L., Allen, D., Lawal, E., Dickson, D., & Denis, A. (2019). Assessing for and managing chronic insomnia in primary care settings. *The Nurse Practitioner, 44*(7), 27–35. doi:10.1097/01.NPR.0000559843.91496.20

Fosnocht, K., & Ende, J. (2019). *Approach to the adult patient with fatigue*. UpToDate. Retrieved from https://www.uptodate.com/contents/approach-to-the-adult-patient-with-fatigue?search=fatigue&source=search_result&selectedTitle=1~150&usage_type=default&display_rank=1

Miller, M. (2019). *Approach to the patient with muscle weakness*. UpToDate. Retrieved from https://www.uptodate.com/contents/approach-to-the-patient-with-muscle-weakness?search=muscle%20weakness%20adult&source=search_result&selectedTitle=1~150&usage_type=default&display_rank=1

Muncie, H., Sirmans, S., & James, E. (2017). Dizziness: Approach to evaluation and management. *American Family Physician, 95*(3), 154–162.

Parmar, J., Dobbs, B., Mc Nay, R., Kirwan, C., Cooper, T., Marin, A., & Gupta, N. (2014). Diagnosis and management of dementia in primary care. *Canadian Family Physician, 60*, 457–465.

12

Practice Essentials for Obstetrics and Gynecology

This journey through the subspecialties progresses with some of the most common complaints that result in the client's visit to the primary care provider—disorders of the gynecological system. Although these conditions may often require specialty consultation with a women's health provider, particularly in the pregnant client, it is often the primary care provider who initiates diagnosis and management. As always, effective management plans can only be developed once the provider has identified the correct condition.

WOMEN'S HEALTH IN PRIMARY CARE

Updates in Contraceptive Technology

Oral Contraceptive Agents

Oral contraception is one of the most common forms of reversible contraception. Products include combination pills containing estrogen and progesterone and progestin-only pills. Products have failure rates of approximately 7.2% to 9% with typical use and are safe for most patients (Brown, Desmukh, & Antell, 2017).

Estrogen-containing contraceptives may increase the risk of venous thromboembolism, so patients with conditions associated with a risk of cardiovascular events should not use oral contraception products that contain estrogen (Brown et al., 2017). Oral contraceptive pills can be prescribed any time if the provider is reasonably certain that the patient is not pregnant, and blood pressure measurement is the only physical examination or testing necessary to conduct prior to prescribing.

There are a number of noncontraceptive benefits of oral contraceptives. These include a reduction in the risk of ovarian and endometrial cancers, more favorable bleeding patterns, and improvement in menstruation-related symptoms, such as acne, hirsutism, migraine headaches, dysmenorrhea, and premenstrual dysphoric disorder (Brown et al., 2017; Evans & Sutton, 2015). These authors also suggest that continuous daily use of oral contraceptive pills and extended (3-month) cycles are reasonable alternatives to monthly use and can further improve menstrual-associated symptoms.

Many products with a range of dosing options are available, and, typically, the lower the prescriber selects, the minimal the anticipated side effects are. Some pearls for practice are described as follows (Stewart & Black, 2015): If clients report nausea, the provider should exclude pregnancy, instruct them to take the pill at night to reduce symptoms, reduce the dose, or eliminate the estrogen.

Similarly, if the client presents complaining of breast tenderness, the provider may elect to reduce the estrogen and/or progestogen dose. When bloating and/or fluid retention is reported, strategies include the reduction of estrogen dose or a product change to progestogen with a mild diuretic effect. Consider extended use of products for clients using oral contraceptive agents who present with headaches during menstruation. Finally, extended pill regimens should be considered for clients who present with dysmenorrhea to reduce the frequency of bleeding, and an alternate form of contraception should be considered when breakthrough bleeding is reported.

Other Contraceptive Products

The intrauterine device (IUD) is one of the most common reversible contraceptive methods worldwide. The IUD is typically safe and highly effective for most women of childbearing age. The IUD is designed for extended use (up to 12 years depending on product type). There are two major types of IUD—hormonal and copper. Some women discontinue use of the copper IUD due to undesirable side effects such as pain, cramping, and heavy bleeding, which typically improve after 6 to 12 months of use (Sanders et al., 2018). Most types make periods lighter and shorter, and some will not menstruate at all while the device is in place.

The insertion of an IUD is a highly specialized procedure with risk. Therefore, only an experienced provider should engage in the practice of IUD insertion due to the risk of uterine perforation. An IUD is to be removed if the client elects to become pregnant or if the duration of recommended device use has been reached. Again, only the trained provider should engage in this practice.

The client with an IUD may present to the primary care setting experiencing one or more of the side effects or adverse reactions listed in Table 12.1.

Table 12.1

Side Effects and Adverse Reactions of IUDs

Potential Side Effects of an IUD	Serious Adverse Reactions of an IUD
Vulvovaginitis	Ectopic pregnancy
Ovarian cyst	Ruptured ectopic pregnancy
Abdominal pain/pelvic pain	Spontaneous abortion
Headache/migraine	Depression
Acne	Uterine perforation
Dysmenorrhea	Pelvic inflammatory disease
Breast pain	Embedded device
Increased bleeding	

IUD, intrauterine device.
Source: Data from ReliasMedia. (2016). *LARC options expand with new intra-uterine device*. Retrieved from https://www.reliasmedia.com/articles/138889-larc-options-expand-with-new-intrauterine-device

As always, a thorough and comprehensive history on the type of device and length of use is crucial. A pelvic ultrasound to determine placement and prompt referral for gynecological and/or emergency services is indicated in the event a serious adverse reaction is suspected. More recently, some types of IUDs are increasingly being used to treat women with endometriosis (Wood, n.d.).

In the past, the IUD was not recommended in women with more than one sexual partner due to the risk of sexually transmitted infection and pelvic inflammatory disease. In recent times, there is growing popularity of this contraception method among groups once considered to be excluded from recommended use, such as college-age women, due to the efficacy and ease of use (Kelsey & Sridhar, 2016). With proper anticipatory guidance provided by the seasoned practitioner, such as unexplained fever, chills, difficulty breathing, severe pelvic pain, abnormal vaginal discharge, or heavy bleeding, this effective form of contraception is a viable option for this population of women where missed pills could result in decreased efficacy of the contraceptive benefit (Planned Parenthood, n.d.).

Emergency Contraception

Clients may present to primary care settings seeking emergency contraceptive services. There are two basic options to be considered. The first is the insertion of a copper IUD within 120 hours after having unprotected intercourse. This is the most effective form of emergency contraception   (https://www.plannedparenthood.org/learn/morning -after-pill-emergency-contraception/which-kind-emergency -contraception-should-i-use). As briefed earlier, only an experienced provider should engage in the practice of IUD insertion due to the risk of uterine perforation.

The second is to take an emergency contraceptive, or morning-after, pill within 120 hours after having unprotected intercourse. There are two types of morning-after pills. The first is ulipristal acetate. Ulipristal acetate requires a prescription and is the most effective type of morning-after pill. Ulipristal acetate is effective if taken up to 120 hours after unprotected intercourse. This agent is less effective if the client weighs more than 195 pounds.

The second morning-after pill option is a pill with levonorgestrel, which can be purchased over the counter. It is important to educate the client that these agents work best when taken within 72 hours after unprotected intercourse. Although they can be taken up to 120 hours, the sooner they are taken, the higher the efficacy. This agent is less effective if the client weighs more than 155 pounds (https://www.planned parenthood.org/learn/morning-after-pill-emergency-contraception/ which-kind-emergency-contraception-should-i-use).

Nausea and vomiting were the main adverse effects associated with emergency contraception. Levonorgestrel users had fewer side effects than those who used other agents. Ulipristal acetate users were more likely to have a menstrual return after the expected date. Copper IUDs were associated with higher risks of abdominal pain than emergency contraceptive pills (Shen, Che, Showell, Chen, & Cheng, 2019).

Updates in Menopause

The management of the perimenopausal and menopausal client poses an array of challenges to the provider in primary care settings. It is typically the women's health provider with expertise in menopause who provides effectively counseling and support. However, the savvy primary care provider recognizes when the complaint may be hormonal in nature and advises accordingly.

For instance, the latest National Institute for Health and Care Excellence guidelines on the diagnosis and management of menopause include the following key messages. The management of estrogen deficiency must be individualized, and follicle-stimulating hormone testing for diagnosis in women older than 45 years should be eliminated. In addition, patient education should include counseling on contraception during menopause, and breast cancer survivors should be provided with all treatment options for menopausal symptoms. Furthermore, the risks and benefits of hormone replacement therapy should be weighed for vasomotor symptoms, and vaginal estrogen can be used on a long-term basis. Also, the ongoing monitoring of symptoms is encouraged during hormone replacement therapy; there are no arbitrary limits for the duration of hormone replacement therapy; and benefits and risks of hormone replacement therapy vary significantly and are strongly influenced by baseline risk and lifestyle factors. Finally, fluoxetine and paroxetine should not be given concurrently with tamoxifen and antidepressants, and clonidine should not be routinely prescribed for menopausal symptoms (http://web.a.ebscohost.com.ezproxy.wpunj.edu/ehost/pdfviewer/pdfviewer?vid=1&sid=d84ffe3f-40a5-4992-84d2-df5dba713d16%40sessionmgr4006).

Complaints Involving the Female Breast

Clients often present to primary care settings with complaints involving the breast. The most common complaints often involve pain/tenderness, swelling, and/or the presence of a palpable lump. Typically, following a thorough history and physical exam, the experienced primary care provider will initiate a thorough workup that would include a mammogram and possibly an ultrasound as well. Other imaging, such as breast MRI, may, in fact, also be indicated, although any abnormalities on a mammogram or ultrasound would be referred to a breast specialist for further diagnostic imaging and, perhaps, a biopsy.

It has been reported that one in eight women in the United States will develop breast cancer in her lifetime and that breast cancer is the most common cancer in American women, except for skin cancers. Death rates from breast cancer have been declining due to better screening and early detection and continually improving treatment options (National Breast Cancer Foundation, n.d.). Therefore, all complaints regarding the breast should be taken under serious consideration and evaluated accordingly.

Women's Health Screening in Primary Care

It is often the primary care practitioner who may be the sole provider of women's health prevention activities. Many clients may not see their women's health provider on a regular basis as recommended, so it is the primary care provider's role to ensure that age-appropriate health maintenance activities have been conducted and are monitored on a regular basis.

Fast Facts

Some integral women's health maintenance screening activities that the skillful primary care provider is careful to incorporate into the management plan include the following:

- Pap smears
- Body mass index
- Blood pressure
- Cholesterol testing
- Blood glucose testing
- Mammography
- Bone density testing
- Dental care
- Skin cancer screening
- Colon cancer screening

PREGNANT PATIENTS IN PRIMARY CARE SETTINGS

It is typically not appropriate for pregnancy to be managed in primary care settings. Although a natural and often healthy state, pregnancy poses a great risk for both the pregnant patient and her fetus. Therefore, only the highly experienced women's health clinician is charged with the management of the pregnant client. There are, however, conditions that the primary care provider may be involved in managing when the pregnant client presents seeking care.

Primary Care Management of the Pregnant Client

Although prenatal care is managed by the client's women's health provider, it is often the primary care provider who is faced with the pregnant client who presents with common conditions in pregnancy. Examples include upper respiratory infection, conjunctivitis, urinary tract infection, vaginitis, dermatitis, and minor sprains or strains. Management principles are typically the same as for a client who is not pregnant. There are, however, a number of pearls for the experienced provider to note before determining management plans.

Often, the women's health provider will provide the pregnant client with a list (or post on their web page) of over-the-counter agents that are acceptable during pregnancy. This is often a good start depending on the primary care need. Acetaminophen is safe at any time during pregnancy, as are most cold medications after the first trimester. Many gastrointestinal medications such as histamine H$_2$ blockers and proton pump inhibitors have not been found to demonstrate significant fetal effects. Nonsteroidal anti-inflammatory drugs are generally not recommended in pregnancy. Topical creams are generally considered safe. All over-the-counter medication use should be discussed with patients, and the effects of the symptoms should be balanced with the risks and benefits of each medication (Servey & Chang, 2014).

Prescription of pharmacological agents can be given in accordance with standard practice guidelines. The A, B, C, D, and X risk categories, in use since 1979, were replaced by the Pregnancy and Lactation Labeling Final Rule that went into effect on June 30, 2015. This new labeling rule provides updated information to help clinicians explain the potential benefits and risks for the mother, fetus, and breastfeeding child. This change was implemented due to a concern expressed by stakeholders that the letter categories were often misinterpreted as a grading system for the risks of a drug, resulting in prescribing decisions based on the category rather than on an understanding of the underlying information (Whyte, n.d.).

Typically, x-rays are avoided during pregnancy; however, with proper shielding of the abdomen, it is possible to conduct an x-ray of the head, teeth, chest, or extremities if the x-ray is necessary for the diagnostician. According to the American College of Radiology, no single diagnostic x-ray has a radiation dose significant enough to cause adverse effects in a developing embryo or fetus. In general, CAT scans are not recommended during pregnancy unless the benefits of the CAT scan clearly outweigh the potential risk (American Pregnancy Association, n.d.). It may be prudent to consult with the client's women's health provider prior to conducting an x-ray if possible.

Exposure to MRI during the first trimester of pregnancy was not associated with increased risk of harm to the fetus or in early childhood. Gadolinium MRI at any time during pregnancy was associated with an increased risk of a broad set of rheumatological, inflammatory, or infiltrative skin conditions and for stillbirth or neonatal death (Ray, Vermeulen, Bharatha, Montanera, & Park, 2016). Overall, MRI may be a safer diagnostic test to consider for the pregnant client.

Updates in Obstetrics

It is common for the primary care provider to diagnose pregnancy. Although over-the-counter pregnancy tests are most often accurate once a menstrual period has been missed, women typically present to primary/urgent care settings for the verification of pregnancy. Urine testing is effective to determine the evidence of pregnancy, yet a blood β-human chorionic gonadotropin is a more accurate means of validating the diagnosis. Once confirmed, the client should be referred for obstetrical care. The first prenatal visit typically takes place around 8 weeks. In addition, the use of prenatal vitamins should be encouraged. Warning signs should be reviewed such as vaginal bleeding, convulsions, severe headaches, fever, severe abdominal pain, fast or difficult breathing, or swelling of fingers, face, and legs (National Center for Biotechnology Information, n.d.).

Fast Facts

- Oral contraceptive pills can be prescribed any time if the provider is reasonably certain that the patient is not pregnant, and blood pressure measurement is the only physical examination or testing necessary to conduct prior to prescribing.
- The popularity of the IUD is growing among groups once considered to be excluded from recommended use, such as college-age women, due to the efficacy and ease of use.
- It is important to educate the clients that the over-the-counter emergency contraceptive agents work best when taken within 72 hours after unprotected intercourse; although they can be taken up to 120 hours—the sooner they are taken, the higher the efficacy.
- The ongoing monitoring of menopausal symptoms is encouraged during hormone replacement therapy; there are no arbitrary limits for the duration of hormone replacement therapy; and benefits and risks of hormone replacement therapy vary significantly and are strongly influenced by baseline risk and lifestyle factors.
- Primary care screening such as Pap smears, body mass index, blood pressure, cholesterol and blood glucose testing, referrals for mammography, bone density testing, and dental care, and skin and colon cancer screening are integral women's health maintenance activities.
- All over-the-counter medication use should be discussed with the pregnant patient, and the effects of the symptoms should be balanced with the risks and benefits of each medication.

(continued)

(*continued*)

- According to the American College of Radiology, no single diagnostic x-ray has a radiation dose significant enough to cause adverse effects in a developing embryo or fetus.
- The newly diagnosed pregnant client should be educated on warning signs to report such as vaginal bleeding, convulsions, severe headaches, fever, severe abdominal pain, fast or difficult breathing, or swelling of fingers, face, and legs.

SUMMARY

This journey through the subspecialties continued with a variety of collaborative clinical practice sessions with physician specialists and nurse practitioners practicing in specialty settings. Clients presented with common complaints that often begin with their visit to the primary care provider who specializes in managing women's health conditions. This clinical immersion experience led to the identification of hot topics that the primary/urgent care nurse practitioner is expected to diagnose or perhaps initiate during the management of female clients. As always, effective management plans can only be developed once the provider has identified the correct etiology.

References

American Pregnancy Association. (n.d.). *CAT scans and pregnancy*. Retrieved from https://americanpregnancy.org/pregnancy-health/cat-scans/

Brown, E., Desmukh, P., & Antell, K. (2017). Contraception update: Oral contraception. *Family Practice Essentials, 462*, 11–19.

Evans, G., & Sutton, E. (2015). Oral contraception. *Medical Clinics of North America, 99*(3), 479–503. doi:10.1016/j.mcna.2015.01.004

Kelsey, R., & Sridhar, A. (2016). Perceived knowledge of intrauterine devices at an Urban University Student Center. *Obstetrics & Gynecology, 127*, 124S. doi:10.1097/01.AOG.0000483504.20004.ed

National Breast Cancer Foundation, Inc. (n.d.). *Breast cancer facts*. Retrieved from https://www.nationalbreastcancer.org/breast-cancer-facts

National Center for Biotechnology Information. (n.d.). *Danger signs in pregnancy*. Retrieved from https://www.ncbi.nlm.nih.gov/books/NBK304178/

Planned Parenthood. (n.d.). *How safe is the IUD?* Retrieved from https://www.plannedparenthood.org/learn/birth-control/iud/how-safe-is-the-iud

Ray, J., Vermeulen, M., Bharatha, A., Montanera, W., & Park, A. (2016). Association between MRI exposure dring pregnancy and fetal and childhood outcomes. *JAMA, 316*(9), 952–961. doi:10.1001/jama.2016.12126

ReliasMedia. (2016). *LARC options expand with new intrauterine device.* Retrieved from https://www.reliasmedia.com/articles/138889-larc-options-expand-with-new-intrauterine-device

Sanders, J., Adkins, D., Kaur, S., Storck, K., Gawron, L., & Turok, D. (2018). Bleeding, cramping, and satisfaction among new copper IUD users: A prospective study. *PLoS One, 13*(11), e0199724. doi:10.1371/journal.pone.0199724

Servey, J., & Chang, J. (2014). Over-the-counter medications in pregnancy. *American Family Physician, 90*(8), 548–555.

Shen, J., Che, Y., Showell, E., Chen, K., & Cheng, L. (2019). Interventions for emergency contraception. *Cochrane Systematic Review – Intervention.* doi:10.1002/14651858.CD001324.pub6

Stewart, M. A., & Black, K. I. (2015). *Choosing a combined oral contraceptive pill.* Retrieved from https://www.semanticscholar.org/paper/Choosing-a-combined-oral-contraceptive-pill.-Stewart-Black/b371ee2da9b4b063d8735f901b4344968a133722/figure/1

Whyte, J. (n.d.). *FDA implements new labeling for medications used during pregnancy and lactation.* Retrieved from https://www.aafp.org/afp/2016/0701/p12.pdf

Wood, R. (n.d.). *Mirena.* Retrieved from https://endometriosis.org/treatments/mirena/

13

Practice Essentials for Ophthalmology

The adult client may present to the primary care setting with a variety of symptoms related to the eye. Although many of these are appropriate for the primary care provider to diagnose and manage, some conditions may be persistent or significant enough to be referred to the ophthalmologist. The skillful provider is knowledgeable on the standards of care for the client with an ophthalmic condition, as well as the red flags to assess and refer for a consultation with the specialty provider.

As always, the skillful primary care practitioner knows that a comprehensive history and thorough examination are critical steps in determining the proper management plan. Box 13.1 presents key elements of the initial client history to be gathered from the client who presents to the primary care setting with a condition of the eye.

BOX 13.1 EYE-RELATED CLIENT HISTORY

Visual changes	Duration of symptoms	Presence of a foreign body
History of trauma	Recent eye surgery	Headache
Nausea	Ocular discharge	Photophobia
Contact use/care	Sandy sensation	Dryness
Tearing	Crusting	Matting

Source: Data from Kaur, S., Larson, H., & Nattis, A. (2019). Primary care approach to eye conditions. *Osteopathic Family Physician, 11*(2), 28–34.

The initial examination of the eye includes inspection of the eyelid, periorbital region, sclera, and conjunctiva including eversion of the upper lid, visual examination using a Snellen chart, and an evaluation using a Wood's lamp to assess for corneal abrasion or foreign body (Kaur et al., 2019). A slit lamp may be used to provide greater magnification in some settings.

HEALTH MAINTENANCE OF THE EYE

Periodic health maintenance activities should also include regular visits to the ophthalmologist for screening. The American Academy of Ophthalmology recommends that adults receive a complete eye examination once they reach the age of 40 years. Adult clients with diabetes, hypertension, and/or a family history of eye disease will need more frequent examinations. As the risk of age-related eye diseases such as cataracts, diabetic retinopathy, age-related macular degeneration, or glaucoma increases over time, by age 65 years, the client will likely need more frequent screening—at least every 1 to 2 years. These recommendations should be provided by the specialist (Turbert, 2018).

CONDITIONS OF THE EYELID

Blepharitis

Clients may also report symptoms of an inflammatory condition of the eyelid margins, such as blepharitis, to the primary care provider. If suspected, the skillful practitioner is certain to evaluate the client for associated conditions such as seborrheic dermatitis or rosacea. Treatment is supportive. The client should be educated on eyelid hygiene, lid massage, and the use of warm compresses. If the client does not respond, topical erythromycin or bacitracin ophthalmic ointment may be considered, and in severe cases, Kaur et al. (2019) recommend the use of oral antibiotics such as doxycycline or tetracycline. A dermatologist may be consulted for difficult-to-manage cases of blepharitis.

Hordeolum

When the client presents with an erythematous, painful abscess of the eyelid, most often the source of the discomfort is a hordeolum. It has been reported that most hordeola resolve spontaneously without intervention, and, typically, a warm compress helps to facilitate drainage and supports healing. There is no evidence to suggest that antibiotics or steroids are useful to treat a hordeolum (Ghosh & Ghosh, 2019).

Chalazion

Additionally, the client may complain of a painless, localized swelling of the eyelid, which is known as a chalazion, or an obstruction of the meibomian glands. Although similar in appearance to the hordeolum, chalazia tend to be painless and less erythematous. Small chalazia will resolve without intervention, whereas larger lesions can be drained using warm compresses. Again, antibiotic therapy is not indicated. Persistent or difficult-to-manage lesions should be evaluated by an ophthalmologist, particularly if unilateral, as a carcinoma must be ruled out (Ghosh & Ghosh, 2019).

CONDITIONS OF THE EYE

Conjunctivitis

One of the most common eye conditions that clients present to the primary care setting with is conjunctivitis. The seasoned provider is careful to differentiate between noninfectious (e.g., allergic, foreign body, or chemical burns) and infectious causes (e.g., viral or bacterial).

Fast Facts

Viral conjunctivitis is often associated with an upper respiratory infection, whereas bacterial conjunctivitis is usually unilateral and consists of a greater amount of mucopurulent secretions, matting upon awakening, and lid swelling than viral conjunctivitis (Kaur et al., 2019).

Antibiotic drops/ointments such as erythromycin, bacitracin, trimethoprim–polymyxin B, sulfacetamide, fluoroquinolone, or azithromycin are effective and well tolerated (Jacobs, 2020). Furthermore, education on comfort measures and prevention of transmission are indicated.

Allergic conjunctivitis is often seen in the client with allergic rhinitis, eczema, or asthma; symptoms include bilateral eye lacrimation, itching, and diffuse erythema (Kaur et al., 2019). Instruction on the avoidance of triggers and symptom management are important components of the plan of care. The pharmacologic management of the client with allergic conjunctivitis includes consideration of the following agents: vasoconstrictor/antihistamine combinations, antihistamines with mast cell-stabilizing properties, mast cell stabilizers, nonsteroidal anti-inflammatory drugs, glucocorticoids, and/or oral antihistamines (Hamrah & Dana, 2019). Although a culture may be useful in determining the cause of persistent conjunctivitis, the client with recurrent or difficult-to-manage symptoms should likely be referred to a specialist for evaluation and management.

Keratoconjunctivitis Sicca

Keratoconjunctivitis sicca, or dry eye, is a condition caused by decreased tear production or poor tear quality. At-risk clients who may present to the primary care setting are typically older females who may report a history of autoimmune conditions, such as rheumatoid arthritis and Sjögren's syndrome (Kaur et al., 2019). Treatment is initiated based on the etiology and severity of symptoms. Initially, the use of artificial tears, nightly lubricant ointments, and a humidifier is recommended. Other treatment options include cyclosporine ophthalmic drops or topical corticosteroids; however, if first-line therapies are proven ineffective, a referral to an ophthalmologist is indicated (Kaur et al., 2019).

Subconjunctival Hemorrhage

The client may present to the primary care setting complaining of a bright red patch in the subconjunctival space that is not painful. Typically, a conjunctival blood vessel has ruptured, resulting in the subconjunctival hemorrhage. Often, no treatment is required. Kaur et al. (2019) describe supportive care as warm compresses and the use of lubricants. However, in the event pain is present, the seasoned provider is suspicious of the presence of a foreign body and/or corneal involvement. Overall, a referral to an ophthalmologist is indicated if there is corneal involvement, a history of blunt trauma, drainage, or persistent pain (Kaur et al., 2019).

Corneal Abrasion

The client who presents to the primary care setting complaining of eye pain with photophobia and/or a sensation of a foreign body should be evaluated for a corneal abrasion, which is evident on fluorescein staining. Once identified, the corneal abrasion is treated with topical antibiotics such as erythromycin, trimethoprim–polymyxin B, or sulfacetamide; ciprofloxacin, ofloxacin, gentamicin, or tobramycin are recommended for contact lens wearers. Discomfort for the mild-to-moderate abrasion is managed with oral nonsteroidal anti-inflammatory drugs, although larger abrasions may require opioid analgesics as they can cause more discomfort and take longer to heal (Jacobs, 2019).

Fast Facts

Corneal abrasions should never be treated with a topical corticosteroid, patching should be reserved for larger abrasions only, and all corneal abrasions should be reevaluated in 24 hours for signs of healing.

As the client with herpes simplex virus keratitis may report eye pain, photophobia, blurred vision, tearing, and redness, the seasoned provider should be careful to distinguish these from those of a corneal abrasion (White & Chodosh, 2014). If symptoms do not improve within 48 hours, the patient should be referred to an ophthalmologist (Kaur et al., 2019).

In the event a high-risk trauma has been reported, such as blunt trauma or injury from a sharp object, the seasoned primary care provider must evaluate for open globe injury, which warrants the avoidance of placing any medication into the eye and prompt emergency referral to an ophthalmologist (Jacobs, 2019). Furthermore, if a foreign body such as sand, dirt, or an eyelash is visualized, it should be removed using an eye flush, but the protruding foreign body in the eye should be left in place with removal deferred to the specialist. Overall, tetanus prophylaxis is warranted for penetrating eye injuries.

Episcleritis

The adult client may also present to the primary care setting complaining of redness, irritation, and watering of the eye with preserved vision (Dana, 2019). Here, a diagnosis of episcleritis, or an inflammation of the superficial layers of the episcleral, is considered (Kaur et al., 2019). This condition is usually self-limiting and will resolve after 2 to 3 weeks. However, further investigation is needed if there are recurrent episodes as, often, the client with an inflammatory disease such as rheumatoid arthritis, systemic lupus erythematosus, Sjögren's syndrome, Lyme disease, or Crohn's disease will complain of symptoms of episcleritis (Dana, 2019). Treatment consists of supportive care and artificial tears, but in some cases, the client may require a short course of topical steroids (Kaur et al., 2019). When a systemic disorder is suspected, referral to a specialist (likely rheumatology) is indicated.

Ptosis

Ptosis is defined as a drooping or falling of the upper eyelid. There are many etiologies of ptosis (Kaur et al., 2019). Although ptosis can be congenital, the adult client may present to the primary care setting complaining of acquired ptosis, where a referral or, perhaps, surgery may be indicated. Possible causes of ptosis include Horner's syndrome, third nerve palsy, aneurysm, tumor, trauma, and myasthenia gravis (Lee, 2018).

Fast Facts

In patients with Horner's syndrome, the classic triad of miosis, ptosis, and anhidrosis is seen, and if Horner's syndrome is suspected, or if diplopia, periorbital pain, and/or a headache is present, an urgent referral to a neurologist and ophthalmologist is warranted (Kaur et al., 2019).

Cataracts

Older adult clients who complain of slowly progressive visual loss must be evaluated for the presence of a cataract or a clouding of the eye's crystalline lens. Related symptoms may include a reduced color perception, monocular diplopia, and nighttime glare (Kaur et al., 2019). This condition is common in the older adult client, and same-day surgical management is rather effective. Therefore, the client must be referred for a consultation, evaluation, and management by an ophthalmologist who performs cataract surgery.

OCULAR EMERGENCIES

It is critical that the primary care provider be familiar with the signs and symptoms of some of the most common ocular emergencies such as uveitis, malignancies, retinal detachment, acute angle-closure glaucoma, globe injuries, or chemical burns (Kaur et al., 2019). If not recognized and treated early in the progression, these can lead to permanent vision loss. Therefore, immediate attention of a specialist is warranted.

Uveitis

Uveitis is an inflammatory condition where the client presents complaining of redness, photophobia, floaters, and pain to the eye, as well as nonocular symptoms such as back pain, joint stiffness, or dysuria. On physical exam, there may be optic disc swelling and edema, conjunctival injection and deposits, floating inflammatory cells and protein, retinal and choroid hemorrhages, exudates, and infiltrates. Although the initial systemic workup for the client with uveitis includes a complete blood count, erythrocyte sedimentation rate, antinuclear antibody, Lyme, rapid plasma reagin, and chest x-ray, all patients with uveitis should be referred to an ophthalmologist within 24 hours for evaluation and management (Kaur et al., 2019; Rosenbaum, 2018).

Malignancies

The primary care provider may first encounter the client with eyelid tumors, and thus should discuss the possible etiologies and refer accordingly. Some common types of malignancies related to the eye with descriptions and management plans are presented in Table 13.1.

Table 13.1

Eye Malignancies and Management Plans		
Basal cell carcinoma	Most common eyelid malignancy Appears in the lower and medial region Pearly nodule in appearance Lashes may be missing if in lid region Low potential to metastasize/locally invasive	Surgical resection Cryotherapy Radiation
Squamous cell carcinoma	Less prevalent More aggressive Erythematous, raised, scaly central ulceration Occurs most frequently on the upper lid Actinic keratosis can be a precursor Metastasizes to the lymph nodes	Surgical resection

(continued)

Table 13.1

Eye Malignancies and Management Plans (*continued*)		
Sebaceous carcinoma	Invades locally and spreads to lymph nodes Occurs in middle-aged to elderly patients May mimic chalazion or blepharitis Aggressive tumor Metastasis to the lungs, liver, and bone	Surgical resection Radiation Chemotherapy

Source: Data from Kaur, S., Larson, H., & Nattis, A. (2019). Primary care approach to eye conditions. *Osteopathic Family Physician, 11*(2), 28–34.

Retinal Detachment

Clients may present to the primary care setting complaining of a sensation of unilateral flashing lights and floaters with or without severe vision loss. Risk factors include increasing age, myopia, traumatic injury, family history, cataract surgery, and a previous retinal detachment in the contralateral eye (Kaur et al., 2019). If retinal detachment is suspected, an immediate referral to an ophthalmologist for evaluation and surgical management is indicated.

Acute Angle-Closure Glaucoma

Any client who presents with unilateral eye pain, headache, nausea, vomiting with a mid-dilated pupil cloudy cornea, and conjunctival injection should be evaluated for acute angle-closure glaucoma. This condition is a medical emergency that can lead to permanent vision loss within hours. Advancing age, female sex, Asian descent, and certain medications (e.g., phenylephrine, ephedrine, or naphazoline) increase a client's risk for acute angle-closure glaucoma (Kaur et al., 2019). Immediate referral is indicated for evaluation and surgical treatment.

Globe Injuries

When the client presents with eye pain, tearing, redness, and decreased vision following blunt trauma to the eye, a globe injury should be considered. Here, the client has suffered a full-thickness rupture through the cornea and sclera (Kaur et al., 2019). This type of injury warrants immediate attention from an ophthalmologist, so prompt referral is indicated.

Chemical Burns

A chemical exposure to the eye often results in an ophthalmologic emergency. Symptoms typically include severe eye pain, redness, tearing, photophobia, and decreased vision. It is important to identify the type and the amount of chemical involved, and a referral to an ophthalmologist for evaluation and management is indicated (Kaur et al., 2019).

Fast Facts

- The treatment of blepharitis includes eyelid hygiene, lid massage, and the use of warm compresses.
- There is no evidence to suggest that antibiotics or steroids are useful to treat a hordeolum.
- The pharmacologic management of the client with allergic conjunctivitis includes consideration of the following agents: vasoconstrictor/antihistamine combinations, antihistamines with mast cell-stabilizing properties, mast cell stabilizers, nonsteroidal anti-inflammatory drugs, glucocorticoids, and/or oral antihistamines.
- Tetanus prophylaxis is warranted for penetrating eye injuries.
- Possible causes of ptosis include Horner's syndrome, third nerve palsy, aneurysm, tumor, trauma, and myasthenia gravis.
- Older adult clients who complain of slowly progressive visual loss, a reduced color perception, monocular diplopia, and nighttime glare must be evaluated for the presence of a cataract.
- The provider must be familiar with the signs and symptoms of some of the most common ocular emergencies and refer accordingly.

SUMMARY

This journey through the subspecialties continued with a collaborative clinical practice session with physician specialists and nurse practitioners practicing in specialty settings. Clients presented with common complaints related to the eye that often begin with their visit to the primary care provider. This clinical immersion experience led to the identification of conditions that the primary care provider is expected to diagnose or perhaps initiate during the management of clients with a variety of ophthalmic conditions. As always, effective management plans can only be developed once the provider has identified the correct etiology. It is further important to include periodic health maintenance screening activities as per recommended guidelines.

References

Dana, R. (2019). *Episcleritis*. UpToDate. Retrieved from https://www.uptodate.com/contents/episcleritis

Ghosh, C., & Ghosh, T. (2019). *Eyelid lesions*. UpToDate. Retrieved from https://www.uptodate.com/contents/eyelid-lesions

Hamrah, P., & Dana, R. (2019). *Allergic conjunctivitis: Management*. UpTo Date. Retrieved from https://www.uptodate.com/contents/allergic-conjunctivitis-beyond-the-basics/print

Jacobs, D. (2019). *Corneal abrasions and corneal foreign bodies: Management*. UpToDate. Retrieved from https://www.uptodate.com/contents/corneal-abrasions-and-corneal-foreign-bodies-management

Jacobs, D. (2020). *Conjunctivitis*. UpToDate. Retrieved from https://www.uptodate.com/contents/conjunctivitis

Kaur, S., Larson, H., & Nattis, A. (2019). Primary care approach to eye conditions. *Osteopathic Family Physician, 11*(2), 28–34.

Lee, M. (2018). *Overview of ptosis*. UpToDate. Retrieved from https://www.uptodate.com/contents/overview-of-ptosis

Rosenbaum, J. (2018). *Uveitis: Etiology, clinical manifestations, and diagnosis*. UpToDate. Retrieved from https://www.uptodate.com/contents/uveitis-etiology-clinical-manifestations-and-diagnosis

Turbert, D. (2018). *Eye exam and vision testing basics*. Retrieved from https://www.aao.org/eye-health/tips-prevention/eye-exams-101

White, M., & Chodosh, J. (2014). *Herpes simplex virus keratitis: A treatment guideline-2014*. Retrieved from https://www.aao.org/clinical-statement/herpes-simplex-virus-keratitis-treatment-guideline

14

Practice Essentials for Orthopedics

This journey through the subspecialties moves on with some of the most common complaints that result in the client's visit to the primary care provider—orthopedic disorders. At times, a referral for diagnostic testing to a specialty provider, such as an orthopedist, or to a rehabilitative specialist, such as physical therapy, is indicated. As always, effective management plans can only be developed once the seasoned provider has identified the correct condition.

ORTHOPEDIC DISORDERS OF THE UPPER BODY

Neck

Neck pain is a common complaint presenting to primary care settings. For most patients, the prognosis is good. The skilled clinician should perform a detailed history and assess for red flags. Some red flags to assess for in the client with neck pain are described in Box 14.1.

It is further critical that a comprehensive neuromuscular examination is conducted and that imaging studies are obtained only when indicated. Treatment includes physical therapy, medications, and in some cases, injections to facilitate an active therapy plan. The goals of treatment are pain reduction and return of daily function. This should include a discharge to an independent home exercise and self-management program (Malanga, Tran, & Maharjan, n.d.).

First-line agents include nonsteroidal anti-inflammatory drugs (NSAIDs) in moderation. Acetaminophen may be used in adjunct in those patients without risk for liver disease. Topical lidocaine or topical NSAIDs may be used in patients with chronic soft tissue pain.

BOX 14.1   NECK PAIN RED FLAGS

Fever	Headache	Photophobia
Trauma	Syncope	Malignancy
Immunodeficiency	Sexual dysfunction	Urinary or fecal retention or incontinence
Ataxia		

Muscle relaxants may be prescribed to reduce muscle spasm, and a short taper of oral steroids may be indicated for acute radicular pain. Opioid analgesics may be tried if no other medication provides relief or others are contraindicated. There are no studies to support the use of anticonvulsants and tricyclic antidepressants in acute neck pain (Malanga et al., n.d.).

Shoulder

Shoulder pain is another common orthopedic complaint clients present to primary care settings for management of. As always, a thorough history is key to proper diagnosis and management. For instance, constant pain suggests inflammation, and pain in other joints suggests the possibility of osteoarthritis or other systemic condition. The skilled clinician is careful to rule out red flags like systemic symptoms such as fever, night sweats, weight loss, or new respiratory symptoms, any abnormality in joint shape, a localized mass or swelling, local erythema, or a hot, tender joint (Artus, Holt, & Rees, 2014). Blood testing may be indicated in the presence of red flags, and plain radiography is usually not initially indicated for non-traumatic shoulder pain of <4 weeks' duration without the presence of red flags. Both ultrasound and MRI can be used for detecting full-thickness rotator cuff tears.

Pain control to return to normal function is the goal of management (Artus et al., 2014). At times, shoulder pain can often be managed with over-the-counter therapies or other nonnarcotic oral analgesics. Opioid use is discouraged unless necessary to achieve pain management goals. Evidence is unclear on the best timing of referral for physical therapy. Although corticosteroid shoulder injection is commonly used, there is no clear evidence for its effectiveness compared with local anesthetic alone, and corticosteroid injections are contraindicated in the presence of acute joint infection or systemic symptoms (Artus et al., 2014).

Elbow, Wrist, and Hand

Elbow pain is another common presenting symptom in primary care settings. After excluding red flags such as swelling and dislocation following trauma, a tender, swollen joint, or rapidly increasing mass, common diagnoses include lateral and medial epicondylitis resulting from a sports injury, manual labor, gripping activities, caring for young children, or other activities of daily living. Reports of elbow stiffness can be associated with conditions of arthritis or trauma. Bilateral elbow pain with stiffness and swelling, limited or loss of full range of motion, the involvement of other joints, and the presence of systemic symptoms suggest inflammatory arthritis. Clients presenting with ulnar nerve radiculopathy may be experiencing medial epicondylitis, osteoarthritis, or inflammatory arthritis. Referred pain from the neck or shoulder region can also present as elbow pain so the assessment of the cervical spine is particularly important in ruling out rheumatoid arthritis. Blood tests are indicated if inflammatory arthritis or gout is suspected, and plain radiographs should be obtained if elbow pain is accompanied by stiffness,which is suggestive of arthritis or trauma. MRI is indicated to diagnose ligament injuries (Javed, Mustafa, Boyle, & Scott, 2015).

Treatment is aimed at alleviating pain and restoring normal physical functioning. Rest, analgesia, and steroid injections provide temporary pain relief, but only as part of a larger treatment plan. The goal of primary care management of tendinopathies includes the avoidance of activities that aggravate symptoms. The management of arthritis includes activity modification, NSAIDs, disease-modifying agents in inflammatory arthritis, steroids, splinting, and use of ice or heat. Physical therapy and corticosteroid injections may also contribute to symptom relief (Javed et al., 2015).

The client with wrist pain often presents to primary care settings. Differentiating between wrist injuries and other conditions of the wrist is the role of the primary care provider. Swelling, tenderness, pain, and edema with a limited range of motion following an injury raise suspicion of a fracture. Pain, paresthesia, numbness, tingling, and weakness in the second, third, and fourth fingers may indicate carpal tunnel syndrome. The risk of carpal tunnel syndrome may be increased in patients with diabetes mellitus, rheumatoid arthritis, osteoarthritis, gout, obesity, or those who are pregnant. Asymptomatic, soft, fluid-filled ganglion cysts can be found on the dorsal surface or volar aspect of the wrist. Pain on the thumb side of the wrist following repetitive injury often indicates de Quervain tenosynovitis (Saccomano & Ferrara, 2017).

A thorough history includes the onset, duration, and location of the pain, sleep disruption, exacerbation of pain with activity, presence of paresthesia, trauma, typical activities performed, occupational history, color changes, history of osteoporosis or osteopenia, and previous attempts at pain management. The skillful provider is certain that the physical assessment includes evaluation for deformity such as that seen in lupus erythematosus or scleroderma and muscle atrophy, which can be indicative of nerve pathology. Nonpharmacologic management includes heat and cold, physical therapy, and/or immobilization. Pharmacologic management typically involves NSAIDs if tolerated, acetaminophen, and/or injectable anesthetics or corticosteroids. Opioid analgesics are used in moderation (Saccomano & Ferrara, 2017). Proper diagnosis is the key to effective management planning.

Clients may present to primary care settings with orthopedic complaints of the hands and fingers. Proper assessment, initial workup, and management strategies are often similar to those acute or chronic conditions previously described related to the shoulder, elbow, and wrist. Hand dominance is an integral part of assessment as is the ruling out of neuropathy or other neurologic symptoms such as weakness or paresthesia. The competent practitioner is aware that symptoms of the hand may indicate neurologic, and not orthopedic, pathology, as patients with a systemic neurological disease can often first present with symptoms and signs affecting the hand (Butler, Murray, & Horwitz, 2016).

Fast Facts

Disorders of the skin and nail, such as paronychia, are important differential diagnoses to consider before determining orthopedic etiology of patient's complaints related to the hand.

ORTHOPEDIC DISORDERS OF THE LOWER BODY

Lower Back

It has been reported that as much as 12% to 28% of the U.S. population has experienced back pain and that it is the leading cause of disability worldwide. More than 90% of cases result from mechanical back pain, and most will resolve with conservative management. Smoking, obesity, a strenuous or sedentary job, low socioeconomic status, job dissatisfaction, and psychological disorders (e.g., depression, psychosis, stress, and sleep disorders) all place the client at increased risk for back pain. The skillful practitioner must distinguish nonspecific back pain from serious systemic etiologies such as cauda equina syndrome, vertebral compression fractures, metastatic cancer, epidural abscess, or osteomyelitis (Badri, Tavakoli, Stefanacci, Langley, & Foster, 2019).

Back pain with normal neurologic examination findings and/ or without radiation to the lower extremities may be related to the inflammation of or damage to the intervertebral disks. Here, management focuses on decreasing inflammation with NSAIDs and physical therapy (Badri et al., 2019).

Assessment should include the location of the pain, whether the pain is constant or intermittent, factors that aggravate or alleviate the symptoms, the presence of bowel or bladder symptoms, and past surgical procedures. Some red flags to assess for in the client with back pain are presented in Box 14.2.

BOX 14.2 BACK PAIN RED FLAGS

Loss of bowel or bladder function	Fever	Unintentional weight loss
Pain that wakes the patient at night	Recent trauma	Bruising/contusion/abrasion
Persistent neurological symptoms	Long-term corticosteroid use	History of osteoporosis

Source: Data from Badri, B., Tavakoli, N., Stefanacci, R., Langley, H., & Foster, K. (2019). Management of back pain in primary care and long-term care settings using a syndrome recognition approach. *Annals of Long-Term Care, 27*(4), 26–31. doi:10.25270/altc.2019.03.00064

Most mechanical back pain will respond to conservative therapy such as cognitive behavioral therapy, physical therapy, and pharmacologic therapy. Short-term opioid therapy may be indicated for more severe pain. Once an initial conservative approach has been attempted, a higher level of care with a more invasive intervention may be considered (Badri et al., 2019). Because of the relationship between back pain and mental health, the seasoned primary care provider is certain to assess mental, as well as physical, health when diagnosing and treating back pain.

Evaluation of the Patient With Hip Pain

Hip pain is a common complaint resulting in a visit to the primary care setting (Wilson & Furukawa, 2014). Anterior hip and groin pain may be associated with osteoarthritis and hip labral tears. Posterior hip pain is often related to conditions such as piriformis syndrome, sacroiliac joint dysfunction, and lumbar radiculopathy. Radiography should be performed if acute fractures, dislocations, or stress fractures are suspected, and MRI should be performed if the history and plain radiograph results are not diagnostic. Magnetic resonance arthrography is the diagnostic test of choice for labral tears (Wilson & Furukawa, 2014).

Fast Facts

Patient age is an important factor in the diagnosis of hip pain. In the adolescent patient, congenital malformations, avulsion fractures, and epiphyseal injuries should be considered. In the adult patient, hip pain is often a result of strains, sprains, a contusion, or bursitis. In the older adult, the skillful practitioner is suspicious for degenerative osteoarthritis or fractures (Wilson & Furukawa, 2014).

Hip labral tears cause groin pain that may radiate to the lateral hip, anterior thigh, and buttock. Typically, an insidious onset is reported, but pain can begin acutely after a traumatic event or in patients with acetabular (hip) dysplasia (Aktan, 2015). Catching or painful clicking with activity may be reported. Magnetic resonance arthrography is considered the diagnostic test of choice for labral tears (Wilson & Furukawa, 2014).

Stress fracture of the hip should be considered if trauma or repetitive weight-bearing exercise is involved. These injuries cause anterior hip or groin pain that is worse with activity. Pain may be present with extremes of motion or hopping. Piriformis syndrome causes buttock pain that is aggravated by sitting or walking. Ischiofemoral impingement leads to nonspecific buttock pain with radiation to the posterior thigh. MRI is useful for the diagnosis (Wilson & Furukawa, 2014).

Knee

The primary care provider is often faced with clients of all ages who complain of knee pain. There is a broad range of diagnoses ranging from acute to chronic conditions.

Fast Facts

Although not always indicated, plain radiographs of the affected knee(s) are often effective in guiding the practitioner toward further management decisions. Often, MRI is an essential element of proper diagnosis and effective corresponding management planning.

The client with osteoarthritis may present to primary care settings complaining of knee pain. Acetaminophen and NSAIDs are typically first-line management agents while a diagnosis is being made and a management plan determined. These can be used alone or in combination with physical therapy to manage most typical causes of chronic knee pain (Jones, Covey, & Sineath, 2015).

The American Academy of Orthopedic Surgeons recommends against the use of glucosamine/chondroitin supplementation for osteoarthritis. Opioid analgesics should only be used when conservative management is deemed ineffective, and weight loss should be encouraged in all patients with osteoarthritis and a body mass index >25. Corticosteroid injections may be an effective management strategy for short-term pain relief in patients with osteoarthritis, and topical NSAIDs may provide relief in clients who do not tolerate the oral form due to gastrointestinal or renal adverse effects. Knee braces may be ineffective for chronic knee pain (Jones et al., 2015). Clients who are candidates for additional therapies and surgical consideration are referred to an orthopedic specialist.

Clients often present to primary care settings following a traumatic injury to the knee. Before a management plan can be developed, it is imperative that the correct diagnosis be determined. Examples include meniscal, tendon, and ligament injuries. Some patients can be managed using a structured exercise physical therapy program, and some will require referral to an orthopedic specialist. Pharmacologic management of pain is indicated. The common practice is to use NSAIDs or acetaminophen. Current guidelines include the avoidance of injecting corticosteroids into weight-bearing tendons. Knee braces can be used to effectively stabilize a traumatic knee ligament or tendon tear, and the client with a full-thickness tear requires immediate referral to an orthopedic surgeon (Jones et al., 2015).

Ankle and Foot

Disorders of the ankle and foot frequently first direct the client to seek care in primary care settings. Acute or chronic pain should be evaluated similarly to those practices described earlier related to hip or knee. What is unique is the evaluation of the injured ankle. Here, the mechanism of injury directs further evaluation and management. More specifically, whether or not the patient can walk after the injury dictates the risk for fracture. Other key elements of assessment include previous injury to the same ankle, as it has been reported that repeat ankle injuries are five times as likely as primary injuries (Maughan, 2019).

The skillful primary care provider conducts an in-depth physical assessment of the painful ankle and foot. This examination focuses upon the presence and location of edema and ecchymosis, as well as palpation of the entire fibula and Achilles tendon. The Ottawa rules are used to guide clinical decision-making and to determine the need for diagnostic imaging following ankle and/or foot trauma. These rules present that plain radiographs of the ankle are only indicated for patients who have pain in the malleolar zone and have bone tenderness at the posterior edge or tip of the lateral or medial malleolus or who are unable to bear weight both immediately after the injury and for four steps in the emergency department or doctor's office. Furthermore, the Ottawa rules dictate that plain radiographs of the foot are only indicated for patients who have pain in the midfoot zone and have bone tenderness at the base of the fifth metatarsal or at the navicular or who are unable to bear weight both immediately after the injury and for four steps in the emergency department or doctor's office. Additionally, if the patient can transfer weight twice to each foot (four steps), they are considered able to bear weight even if they limp (Stiell, n.d.). In general, when there is no swelling or ecchymosis, the physical examination does not elicit pain, and the Ottawa criteria for imaging are not met, there is unlikely to be structural damage of the ankle or foot (Maughan, 2019).

Initial management of the ankle and foot is aimed at the goals to limit pain and swelling and maintain range of motion before gradually increasing exercise. Rest, ice, compression, and elevation (RICE) is recommended for the first 2 to 3 days, although the data on the effectiveness of RICE alone are lacking. Both oral and topical NSAIDs or acetaminophen have been found to be effective. Exercise is the mainstay of recovery from an ankle sprain, and exercises should be started early to maintain range of motion. Grade 1 sprains can be treated with an elastic wrap, and grade 2 sprains can be managed by an elastic wrap and an Aircast. Immobilization with a cast or strict nonweight bearing with an elastic wrap and an Aircast may be necessary in more severe sprains (grade 3). Referral to an orthopedic surgeon is indicated in cases of fracture, dislocation or subluxation, syndesmosis injury, tendon rupture, wound penetrating into the joint, chronic ankle instability, uncertainty of diagnosis, or neurovascular compromise requiring emergency evaluation (Maughan, 2019).

Fast Facts

- Muscle relaxants may be prescribed to reduce muscle spasm, and a short taper of oral steroids may be indicated for acute radicular neck pain.
- Although corticosteroid shoulder injection is commonly used to manage acute shoulder pain, there is no clear evidence for its effectiveness compared with local anesthetic alone.
- The treatment of elbow pain is aimed at alleviating pain and restoring normal physical functioning.
- A thorough history includes the onset, duration, and location of wrist pain, sleep disruption, exacerbation of pain with activity, presence of paresthesia, trauma, typical activities performed, occupational history, color changes, history of osteoporosis or osteopenia, and previous attempts at pain management.
- Patients with a systemic neurological disease can often first present with symptoms and signs affecting the hand.
- Smoking, obesity, a strenuous or sedentary job, low socio-economic status, job dissatisfaction, and psychological disorders (e.g., depression, psychosis, stress, and sleep disorders) all place the client at increased risk for back pain.
- Patient age is an important factor in the diagnosis of hip pain.
- Current guidelines include the avoidance of injecting corticosteroids into weight-bearing tendons of the knee.
- When there is no swelling or ecchymosis, the physical examination does not elicit pain, and the Ottawa criteria for imaging are not met, there is unlikely to be structural damage of the ankle or foot.

SUMMARY

This journey through the subspecialties continued with a variety of collaborative clinical practice sessions with physician specialists and nurse practitioners practicing in specialty settings. Clients presented with common complaints that often begin with their visit to the primary care and resulted in a referral to the orthopedic specialist. This clinical immersion experience led to the identification of hot topics that the primary/urgent care nurse practitioner is expected to diagnose or perhaps initiate during the management of clients with orthopedic conditions. As always, effective management plans can only be developed once the provider has identified the correct etiology.

References

Aktan, N. (2015). Diagnosis and management of acetabular dysplasia in the primary care setting. *The Nurse Practitioner, 39*(8), 9–11. doi:10.1097/01.NPR.0000451881.85908.6a

Artus, M., Holt, T. A., & Rees, J. (2014). The painful shoulder: An update on assessment, treatment, and referral. *British Journal of General Practice, 64*(626), e593–e595. Retrieved from https://bjgp.org/content/64/626/e593

Badri, B., Tavakoli, N., Stefanacci, R., Langley, H., & Foster, K. (2019). Management of back pain in primary care and long-term care settings using a syndrome recognition approach. *Annals of Long-Term Care, 27*(4), 26–31. doi:10.25270/altc.2019.03.00064

Butler, D., Murray, A., & Horwitz, M. (2016). Hand manifestations of neurological disease: Some alternatives to consider. *British Journal of General Practice, 66*(647), 331–332. doi:10.3399/bjgp16X685549

Javed, M., Mustafa, S., Boyle, S., & Scott, F. (2015). Elbow pain: A guide to assessment and management in primary care. *British Journal of General Practice, 65*(640), 610–612. Retrieved from https://www.ncbi.nlm.nih.gov/pmc/articles/PMC4617264/

Jones, B., Covey, C., & Sineath, M. (2015). Nonsurgical management of knee pain in adults. *American Family Physician, 92*(10), 875–883.

Malanga, G. A., Tran, J., & Maharjan, S. S. (n.d.). *Neck pain: Diagnosis and management.* Retrieved from https://www.practicalpainmanagement.com/pain/spine/neck-pain-diagnosis-management

Maughan, K. (2019). *Ankle sprain.* Retrieved from https://www.uptodate.com/contents/ankle-sprain

Saccomano, S., & Ferrara, L. (2017). Assessment and management of wrist pain. *The Nurse Practitioner, 42*(8), 15–19. doi:10.1097/01.NPR.0000520834.99158.4e

Stiell, I. (n.d.). *The Ottawa ankle rules.* Retrieved from http://www.theottawarules.ca/ankle_rules

Wilson, J., & Furukawa, M. (2014). Evaluation of the patient with hip pain. *American Family Physician, 89*(1), 27–34.

15

Practice Essentials for Otolaryngology

Clients often seek care in primary care settings for symptoms related to the ears, nose, and throat. At times, this is appropriate, and a diagnosis can be made and symptoms managed with optimal outcomes achieved. More severe, persistent, or difficult-to-control conditions may often require referral to a specialist in otolaryngology.

EAR

Clients frequently present to primary care settings complaining of ear pain, pressure, drainage, ringing, or hearing loss. As always, a thorough history and focused exam are the keys to effective diagnosis and management. The following presentation focuses on the adult client with ear pain.

Otitis Media

The skilled clinician is proficient in the management of acute otitis media and otitis media with effusion. In the pediatric client with acute otitis media who presents with less severe symptoms, observation for 48 hours may be considered. However, as acute otitis media is not so common in adults, and complications may be significant, current guidelines are to treat all adult clients with antibiotic therapy (Limb, Lustiq, & Durand, 2019).

If a decision is made to treat, amoxicillin–clavulanate is the first-line antibiotic of choice due to the high incidence of resistance. Cefdinir, cefpodoxime, cefuroxime, or ceftriaxone is recommended in clients who are penicillin allergic, but with no known sensitivity to a cephalosporin and doxycycline; azithromycin and clarithromycin are the suggested therapies in those who are allergic to penicillin and cephalosporins (Limb et al., 2019). As the pain can be significant, most adult clients can be managed with a nonsteroidal anti-inflammatory medication or acetaminophen.

Fast Facts

Untreated, acute otitis media can lead to complications. Examples include perforation of the eardrum, tympanosclerosis, mastoiditis, meningitis, and even hearing loss (American Academy of Otolaryngology, 2011).

As antibiotic therapy is not typically indicated in clients who present with otitis media with effusion, the seasoned provider may decide to treat with a short course of oral or topical nasal steroids. Unilateral otitis media with effusion in the adult client with recent onset in origin should prompt an examination of the nasopharynx. Often, the only sign of early nasopharyngeal carcinoma is unilateral otitis media with effusion so, when in question, referral to an otolaryngologist is indicated (American Academy of Otolaryngology, 2011).

Purulent ear drainage in the setting of acute otitis media is likely due to a perforation of the tympanic membrane, and the recommended management is similar to that described for acute otitis media. The evidence is mixed regarding adding a topical antibiotic ear drop without any known autotoxicity such as ciprofloxacin or ofloxacin in clients with a ruptured tympanic membrane over treating with oral antibiotics alone (Limb et al., 2019). Most commonly, the perforation will heal on its own within 2 weeks; however, persistent perforations may require surgical repair so it is often prudent to consult with a specialty provider to reduce the risk of complication (American Academy of Otolaryngology, 2011).

Otitis Externa

Infectious, allergic, and dermatologic disease of the ear may all lead to external otitis, although acute bacterial infection is the most common cause (Goguen, 2018). According to Goguen (2018), the current guidelines for otitis externa are given in Table 15.1.

Table 15.1

Otitis Externa Guidelines	
Mild disease	■ A topical preparation combination such as acetic acid–hydrocortisone (an acidifying agent and a glucocorticoid)
Moderate disease	■ A topical preparation combination that is acidic and contains an antibiotic and a glucocorticoid such as Cipro HC or Cortisporin
Severe disease	■ A topical therapy (as in moderate disease), wick placement, and, if there is evidence of deep tissue infection, oral antibiotics such as ciprofloxacin or ofloxacin

Source: Data from Goguen, L. (2018). *External otitis: Pathogenesis, clinical features, and diagnosis*. UpToDate. Retrieved from https://www.uptodate.com/contents/external-otitis-treatment

It is further important to note that the primary care client who presents with mild-to-moderate external otitis does not need a culture of the ear canal prior to starting antibiotic therapy; however, cultures should be performed in those with severe external otitis, recurrent external otitis, and chronic otitis externa, in immunosuppressed patients, in patients with infections after ear surgery, and in clients who do not respond to initial therapy (Goguen, 2018).

Hearing Loss

Clients may also report hearing loss to the primary care provider. Hearing loss can be caused by a variety of factors. Patients may present with the complaint of being unable to hear, or, commonly, a family member may bring the client for consultation due to difficulty with communication. An effective management plan will, of course, be determined based on the correct diagnosis of the etiology of the symptoms and whether the symptoms are related to conductive or sensorineural hearing loss (see Table 15.2).

Table 15.2

Symptoms of Conductive and Sensorineural Hearing Loss

Conductive hearing loss	■ Cerumen impaction
	■ Swelling of the external auditory canal
	■ Tympanic membrane perforations
	■ Middle ear fluid
	■ Recurrent infections
	■ Trauma
	■ Previous surgery
Sensorineural hearing loss	■ Result of persistent noise exposure
	■ Age-related changes of the eighth cranial nerve (presbycusis)
	■ Genetic factors
	■ Infectious or postinflammatory processes
	■ Acoustic neuroma

Source: Data from American Academy of Otolaryngology—Head and Neck Surgery Foundation. (2011). *Primary care otolaryngology*. Retrieved from https://www.entnet.org/sites/default/files/Oto-Primary-Care-WEB.pdf

Following an assessment of client history and a focused physical examination, audiometry is used to assess a client's hearing level. Clients with abnormal audiometry will typically be referred to an ear, nose, and throat specialist and/or audiologist for management. Furthermore, it is important to note that sudden sensorineural hearing loss is an emergency and requires emergency management. Finally, the prevention of hearing loss is a critical part of client education, and the use of hearing protection for noise avoidance should be part of routine health maintenance (American Academy of Otolaryngology, 2011).

Tinnitus

Adult and older clients may present to primary care settings complaining of tinnitus, which may be described as unilateral or bilateral ringing, buzzing, humming, whistling, hissing, chirping, or "crickets" in the ears. Tinnitus can affect both physical and psychological well-being, interfering with the quality of life (Wu, Cooke, Eitutis, Simpson, & Beyea, 2018). Usually a manifestation of hearing loss, tinnitus may also have other causes such as chronic noise exposure, acoustic trauma, Meniere disease, ototoxic medications, poor sleep, excessive use of caffeine or alcohol, arterial bruits, systemic hypertension, arteriovenous malformation, aneurysms, idiopathic intracranial hypertension, and vascular ear tumors (American Academy of Otolaryngology, 2011; Wu et al., 2018).

Key areas of the history include an assessment of the history of acoustic trauma, occupational noise exposure, or ototoxic medication use, and physical assessment must include a cranial nerve examination and otoscopy; evaluation for signs of infection, eardrum perforation, or middle ear tumors; auscultation for bruits; and referral for audiologic testing. Laboratory testing is typically not indicated, and a magnetic resonance angiogram, venogram of the brain and neck, and/or MRI of the internal auditory canals can be considered as part of the workup (Wu et al., 2018). As always, consultation with a specialty provider may be indicated. More specifically, when tinnitus is pulsatile or unilateral in nature, or if abnormal otoscopy findings are noted, referral to an otolaryngologist is recommended (Wu et al., 2018).

Wu et al. (2018) also describe the principles of tinnitus management. Conservative management includes lifestyle changes to improve sleep, decrease stress levels, and reduce caffeine/alcohol consumption. Other recommendations include the use of hearing aids, white noise machines, and other types of background noise such as a fan or music at bedtime. Melatonin has been shown to improve symptoms, and patients with preexisting anxiety and depression have reported a reduction in tinnitus symptoms with the use of tricyclic antidepressants and selective serotonin reuptake inhibitors. Other treatment options include cognitive behavioral therapy or tinnitus retraining therapy.

Foreign Body

Although less common in adult clients, the occasional adult client may present to the primary care setting complaining of a foreign body inside the ear, such as an insect, Q-tip, bead, or toilet paper. Some contraindications to removal are related to the cooperativeness of the patient, type of foreign body, location in the external auditory canal, and lack of appropriate tools. Curettes, alligator forceps, plain forceps, and irrigation are common options for removal. However, if one or two attempts for removal have been unsuccessful, the client should be referred to an ear, nose, and throat specialist for further management (Lotterman & Sohal, 2019).

NOSE

Clients frequently present to primary care settings complaining of nasal symptoms such as rhinorrhea, postnasal drainage, obstruction, or pain. As always, a thorough history and focused exam are the keys to effective diagnosis and management. The following presentation focuses on the adult client.

Rhinitis

A diagnosis of rhinitis is made when the client presents complaining of congestion, rhinorrhea, sneezing, nasal itching, and/or nasal obstruction, and it is the role of the skillful provider to determine whether the rhinitis should be classified as allergic (related to an allergen) or nonallergic (in relation to nonallergic and noninfectious triggers, e.g., change in the weather, exposure to caustic odors or cigarette smoke, barometric pressure differences) and then to determine the appropriate management plan (Tran, Vickery, & Blaiss, 2011; see Table 15.3).

Table 15.3

Management Plans for Allergic and Nonallergic Rhinitis	
Allergic rhinitis	■ Allergen avoidance ■ Antihistamines (oral and intranasal) ■ Intranasal corticosteroids ■ Intranasal chromones ■ Leukotriene receptor antagonists ■ Immunotherapy ■ Occasional systemic corticosteroids (oral and topical) ■ Occasional decongestants (oral and topical)
Nonallergic rhinitis	■ Intranasal corticosteroids ■ Topical antihistamines ■ Topical anticholinergics such as ipratropium bromide (0.03%) nasal spray ■ Adjunct therapy may include decongestants ■ Adjunct therapy may include nasal saline

Source: Data from Tran, N. P., Vickery, J., & Blaiss, M. S. (2011). Management of rhinitis: Allergic and nonallergic. *Allergy, Asthma & Immunology Research, 3*(3), 148–156. doi:10.4168/aair.2011.3.3.148

As the economic burden is great between direct medical costs and indirect costs such as missed work/school, it is critical that the primary care provider be competent in the diagnosis and management of rhinitis and that management planning incorporate comprehensive education on proper care including the avoidance of triggers (Tran et al., 2011).

Acute Viral Rhinosinusitis

The common cold, or acute viral rhinosinusitis, results in frequent visits to the primary care setting. Common symptoms include low-grade fever, facial discomfort, and purulent nasal drainage. Management is purely symptomatic and may include antipyretic therapy, hydration, analgesics, and decongestants as needed (American Academy of Otolaryngology, 2011). Antibiotic treatment is discouraged. The role of the seasoned provider is to provide client education, which includes the likelihood that spontaneous resolution will occur in approximately 7 to 10 days, as well as the factors leading to appropriate antibiotic use and the risk of antibiotic resistance with inappropriate use.

Acute Bacterial Rhinosinusitis

Acute bacterial rhinosinusitis, or acute sinusitis, may result from prolonged mucosal edema. Here, the client presents to the primary care setting with facial pressure/pain, facial congestion/fullness, purulent nasal discharge, nasal obstruction, and/or anosmia and may also complain of headache, fever, fatigue, cough, toothache, halitosis, and/or ear fullness/pressure. Symptoms that persist beyond 7 to 10 days, or worsen after 5 days, suggest bacterial infection (American Academy of Otolaryngology, 2011).

Symptoms of acute rhinosinusitis persist for <1 month, whereas subacute rhinosinusitis lasts for 1 to 3 months, and chronic sinusitis persists for >3 months. Treatment for acute rhinosinusitis involves a 10-day course of either amoxicillin or trimethoprim/sulfamethoxazole. It may be prudent to consider the use of amoxicillin/clavulanate or a second-generation cephalosporin, macrolide, or quinolone antibiotic as the first-line therapy due to the possibility of resistance to other first-line agents (American Academy of Otolaryngology, 2011).

Fast Facts

Adjunct therapies such as topical decongestants (oxymetazoline) for 3 days, mucolytics (guaifenesin), and oral decongestants may be considered to manage symptoms of acute rhinosinusitis, and severe or recurrent cases may require systemic steroids, but antihistamines and topical steroids are not usually indicated unless there is suspicion of a related allergy.

A referral to a specialty provider may be indicated for persistent infections that do not respond to therapy and/or difficult-to-manage or severe symptoms of rhinosinusitis (e.g., severe pain, orbital cellulitis, or abscess), the presence of three to four episodes of infection per year, or fungal sinusitis that may be compromised by diabetes and likely will require surgery (American Academy of Otolaryngology, 2011).

Nasal Obstruction

Adult clients may present to primary care settings with a complaint of a nasal obstruction such as a septal deviation. Here, clients may present with symptoms such as nasal obstruction, sinusitis, headaches, snoring, and/or obstructive sleep apnea. Typically, a referral to otolaryngology is indicated, as surgery will likely be considered (American Academy of Otolaryngology, 2011).

A nasal foreign body is another possible cause of nasal obstruction. Although a nasal foreign body is a complaint more commonly seen in pediatric settings, the occasional adult client presents to the primary care setting with a foreign body lodged in the nasal cavity. Typically, a referral to a specialist is indicated if the object cannot be easily removed in the primary care setting.

Nasal polyps are an additional frequent cause of nasal obstruction. As 50% of clients who have polyps also have allergies, these individuals should be evaluated for allergies (American Academy of Otolaryngology, 2011). It has been reported that polyps typically respond well to systemic steroids followed by continuous intranasal steroid sprays; however, surgery may be indicated if the symptoms reoccur frequently or do not respond to traditional therapies. Furthermore, the skillful provider is aware that unilateral nasal polyps may be a manifestation of a neoplasm and must be referred to an otolaryngologist for evaluation (American Academy of Otolaryngology, 2011).

Another relatively frequent cause of nasal blockage is rhinitis medicamentosa, which develops when clients repeatedly use decongestant nasal sprays over a long period. Here, the rebound effect causes them to need the spray just to breathe. Management involves the discontinuation of the decongestant spray, while symptoms can be reduced by intranasal steroid spray accompanied by short bursts of systemic steroids (American Academy of Otolaryngology, 2011). Cocaine abuse can also result in this condition, so acquiring a careful history of substance abuse is the role of the seasoned primary care provider. Other causes of nasal obstruction where referral is indicated include intranasal masses such as pyogenic granuloma, Wegner's granulomatosis, sarcoidosis, and neoplasms (American Academy of Otolaryngology, 2011).

THROAT

Clients frequently present to primary care settings complaining of a sore throat. Sore throats are typically caused by a viral or bacterial infection. Some other less common but more serious infections can cause a sore throat, including mononucleosis, influenza, *Neisseria gonococcus*, and HIV. Some noninfectious causes include allergic rhinitis or sinusitis, gastroesophageal reflux disease, smoking or exposure to secondhand smoke, exposure to dry winter air, trauma (e.g., tracheal intubation), vocal strain, medication use (e.g., angiotensin-converting enzyme inhibitors and some chemotherapeutics), and autoimmune disorders (e.g., Kawasaki disease; Chow & Doron, 2019). More urgent symptoms requiring emergent care are presented in Box 15.1 (Chow & Doron, 2019; Stead, 2019).

BOX 15.1 URGENT SYMPTOMS RELATED TO THE THROAT

Dyspnea	Retractions
Tripod position	
Difficulty breathing	Swelling of the neck or tongue
Skin rash	Stiff neck or difficulty opening the mouth
Drooling because unable to swallow	Underlying chronic illness/medication that may impair the immune system
Muffled voice	Hoarseness
Stridor	Tachypnea

Source: Data from Chow, A., & Doron, S. (2019). *Evaluation of acute pharyngitis in adults.* UpToDate. Retrieved from https://www.uptodate.com/contents/evaluation-of-acute-pharyngitis-in-adults; Stead, W. (2019). *Patient education: Sore throat in adults (Beyond the Basics).* UpToDate. Retrieved from https://www.uptodate.com/contents/sore-throat-in-adults-beyond-the-basics

Group A streptococcal pharyngitis should be considered in clients who present with a sudden onset of the sore throat, fever, tonsillopharyngeal and/or uvular edema, patchy tonsillar exudates, cervical lymphadenitis (often tender and anterior), scarlatiniform skin rash and/or strawberry tongue, and/or history of exposure (Chow & Doron, 2019). Antibiotic treatment is recommended for clients with symptomatic pharyngitis or tonsillopharyngitis and a positive rapid antigen test or culture. Oral penicillin or amoxicillin is the first-line drug of choice, whereas cephalosporins, clindamycin, and macrolides are alternatives (Pichichero, 2019).

Fast Facts

- As acute otitis media is not so common in adults, and complications may be significant, current guidelines are to treat all adult clients with antibiotic therapy.
- Cultures should be performed in those with severe external otitis, recurrent external otitis, and chronic otitis externa, in immunosuppressed patients, in patients with infections after ear surgery, and in clients who do not respond to initial therapy.
- Sudden sensorineural hearing loss is an emergency and requires emergency management.
- Conservative management of tinnitus includes lifestyle changes to improve sleep, decrease stress levels, and reduce caffeine/alcohol consumption.
- As the economic burden is great, it is critical that the primary care provider is competent in the diagnosis and management of rhinitis and that management planning incorporates comprehensive education on proper care, including the avoidance of triggers.
- A referral to a specialty provider may be indicated for persistent infections that do not respond to therapy and/or difficult-to-manage or severe symptoms of rhinosinusitis (e.g., severe pain, orbital cellulitis, or abscess), the presence of three to four episodes of infection per year, or fungal sinusitis that may be compromised by diabetes and likely will require surgery.
- Unilateral nasal polyps may be a manifestation of a neoplasm and must be referred to an otolaryngologist for evaluation.
- Group A streptococcal pharyngitis should be considered in clients who present with a sudden onset of the sore throat, fever, tonsillopharyngeal and/or uvular edema, patchy tonsillar exudates, cervical lymphadenitis (often tender and anterior), scarlatiniform skin rash and/or strawberry tongue, and/or history of exposure.

SUMMARY

This journey through the subspecialties continued with a collaborative clinical practice session with physician specialists and nurse practitioners practicing in specialty settings. Clients presented with common complaints of the ears, nose, and throat that often begin with their visit to the primary care provider. This clinical immersion experience led to the identification of conditions that the primary care provider is expected to diagnose or perhaps refer to a specialist in otolaryngology. As always, effective management plans can only be developed once the provider has identified the correct etiology.

References

American Academy of Otolaryngology—Head and Neck Surgery Foundation. (2011). *Primary care otolaryngology.* Retrieved from https://www.entnet.org/sites/default/files/Oto-Primary-Care-WEB.pdf

Chow, A., & Doron, S. (2019). *Evaluation of acute pharyngitis in adults.* UpToDate. Retrieved from https://www.uptodate.com/contents/evaluation-of-acute-pharyngitis-in-adults

Goguen, L. (2018). *External otitis: Pathogenesis, clinical features, and diagnosis.* UpToDate. Retrieved from https://www.uptodate.com/contents/external-otitis-treatment?search=external%20otitis&source=search_result&selectedTitle=1~30&usage_type=default&display_rank=1

Limb, C., Lustiq, L., & Durand, M. (2019). *Acute otitis media in adults.* UpToDate. Retrieved from https://www.uptodate.com/contents/acute-otitis-media-in-adults/print

Lotterman, S., & Sohal, M. (2019). *Ear foreign body removal.* Retrieved from https://www.ncbi.nlm.nih.gov/books/NBK459136/

Pichichero, M. (2019). *Treatment and prevention of streptococcal pharyngitis.* UpToDate. Retrieved from https://www.uptodate.com/contents/treatment-and-prevention-of-streptococcal-pharyngitis?search=streptococcal%20pharyngitis&source=search_result&selectedTitle=1~97&usage_type=default&display_rank=1

Stead, W. (2019). *Patient education: Sore throat in adults (Beyond the Basics).* UpToDate. Retrieved from https://www.uptodate.com/contents/sore-throat-in-adults-beyond-the-basics

Tran, N. P., Vickery, J., & Blaiss, M. S. (2011). Management of rhinitis: Allergic and nonallergic. *Allergy, Asthma & Immunology Research, 3*(3), 148–156. doi:10.4168/aair.2011.3.3.148

Wu, V., Cooke, B., Eitutis, S., Simpson, M., & Beyea, J. (2018). Approach to tinnitus management. *Canadian Family Physician, 64*(7), 491–495.

16

Practice Essentials for Pediatrics

The experienced provider is aware that care is provided to pediatric/adolescent patients and takes principles of development into consideration. For instance, it may be prudent not to wear a lab coat in settings where younger children may be anxious when approached. Furthermore, one might auscultate before performing more invasive techniques (e.g., inspection of the ears or throat) to minimize crying. Finally, the competent nurse practitioner (NP) interviews the adolescent client with the caretaker present and then politely asks the caretaker to step out of the room to ascertain that data collected with them present are, in fact, accurate and complete.

CARE OF INFANTS AND TODDLERS IN PRIMARY CARE SETTINGS

Feeding, Sleeping, and Toileting

Issues related to feeding, sleeping, and toileting are likely the most common complaints that lead to a visit to the pediatric primary care provider. A comprehensive history is an important first step to management. A tired, anxious, or overwhelmed caretaker is looking to the provider to listen and guide them through what may be challenging phases of their child's development. Additionally, with a rise in obesity in the pediatric population, it is crucial that children and caretakers be cognizant of how early eating habits can affect children's health as they develop.

Breast Is Best

The World Health Organization's (WHO) recommendation includes that women should be encouraged and supported to exclusively breastfeed for approximately the first 6 months of life and continue through the first year as age-appropriate complementary foods are introduced. This statement is supported by the American Academy of Pediatrics, the American College of Obstetricians and Gynecologists, the Academy of Breastfeeding Medicine, the Academy of Nutrition and Dietetics, and the Obesity Society. There are numerous benefits including reduced morbidity and mortality, and breastfed infants have a 12% to 24% reduction in the future risk of being overweight or obese (Oken, Fields, Lovelady, & Redman, 2017; see Box 16.1 for some additional benefits of breastfeeding).

BOX 16.1   BREASTFEEDING BENEFITS

Protection against eczema and allergens	Less diarrhea and constipation
Reduced risk of viruses	Decreased urinary tract infections
Minimized ear infections	Less frequent respiratory infections
Protection from inflammatory bowel disease	Reduced likelihood of gastroenteritis
Decreased risk of SIDS	

SIDS, sudden infant death syndrome.

Source: Data from La Leche League International. (n.d.). *Breastfeeding info A to Z*. Retrieved from https://www.llli.org/breastfeeding-info/

The pediatric primary care provider should support parents who elect to exclusively breastfeed, as well as those who supplement with formula to breastfeed as much as they are comfortable doing. It is important that we provide new parents with the current science and refer them to evidence-based patient information resources.

Back to Sleep

Sleep safety must remain the priority of education that takes place during well-child visits. The latest guidelines include that infants are placed on their backs to sleep until the age of 1 year on a flat, firm surface such as a crib or bassinet, which is free from sleep positioners, bumpers, loose bedding, and toys (March of Dimes, 2019). Infants may sleep in the same room as a parent, but not in the same bed. It is also important to be certain that the crib or bassinet is away from hanging window cords or electrical wires and that the room is kept at a comfortable temperature (March of Dimes, 2019). Furthermore, pacifiers may be introduced around 3 to 4 weeks of age, and swaddling may help promote sleep, but rolling is prohibited and should be discontinued by the age of 2 months. Finally, it is imperative that children always sleep in areas that are smoke free (American Family Physician, 2017).

Toileting

Difficulty with elimination can be a challenge for children and their families. Patients present to pediatric primary care settings with a variety of conditions related to elimination, such as gas, constipation, diarrhea, stool withholding, and bedwetting. In addition, caregivers desire support in determining readiness for and strategies for successful toilet training. Some children may be ready to toilet-train as young as 18 months, whereas others require more time in order to be developmentally ready. Caregivers need guidance in recognizing the physiological, cognitive, and verbal signs of toilet training readiness and should be educated on the process of supporting children to toilet-train at the appropriate time using effective strategies for success (Wolraich, 2016).

Probiotic use can be recommended as an effective therapy in reducing the duration of acute infectious diarrhea and antibiotic-associated diarrhea, among other conditions such as colic, constipation, and acid reflux (Sung et al., 2013). In addition, evidence has demonstrated that probiotics were better than placebo in reducing the incidence and duration of upper respiratory tract infections in study participants. Antibiotic use and school absence due to colds were also found to be reduced when pediatric probiotic therapy was introduced (Hao, Dong, & Wu, 2015).

Screen Time

Caregivers will often seek education on social habits and parenting guidelines from the pediatric primary care provider. One common example is the healthy allowance of screen time. Box 16.2 includes the current guidelines according to the American Academy of Pediatrics.

BOX 16.2 AMERICAN ACADEMY OF PEDIATRICS MEDIA USE RECOMMENDATIONS FOR CHILDREN

- The avoidance of screen media other than video-chatting for children under 18 months.
- From 18 to 24 months, watching high-quality programming with children is encouraged.
- Screen time should be limited to 1 hr per day for children aged 2 to 5 years.
- For children aged 6 years and older, consistent limits must be placed on screen time ensuring that media does not take the place of adequate sleep, physical activity, and other healthy lifestyle behaviors.

Source: Data from American Academy of Pediatrics. (2016). *American Academy of Pediatrics announces new recommendations for children's media use*. Retrieved from https://www.aap.org/en-us/about-the-aap/aap-press-room/Pages/American-Academy-of-Pediatrics-Announces-New-Recommendations-for-Childrens-Media-Use.aspx

It is the role of the pediatric/family primary care provider to reinforce these guidelines on a clear and consistent basis during well-child visits.

CARE OF PRESCHOOL- AND SCHOOL-AGED CHILDREN IN PRIMARY CARE SETTINGS

Preschool- and school-aged children present to primary care settings with many of the same conditions, such as acute episodic illness and chronic conditions, that younger and older children do. There are, however, a number of complaints that may be unique to or arise in this population of children. For instance, the rise in mental health issues related to increased usage of social media platforms and resultant bullying behaviors is a challenge the provider in pediatric primary care settings will face.

Fast Facts

Approximately one in five children meet the criteria for a mental health disorder. Of these, anxiety disorders are the most common (13%), followed by attention deficit hyperactivity disorder (7%) and depression (3%; Bostic & Cullins, 2019).

Bullying

School bullying is not a new phenomenon. Over 40 years of research have led to a number of key conclusions for the pediatric primary care provider to be aware of. Hymel and Swearer (2015) report that bullying is evident as early as preschool and peaks during middle school. It takes many forms such as verbal taunts and threats, exclusion, humiliation, rumor spreading, electronic harassment, and direct physical harm, and, currently, 10% to 33% of students report victimization by peers. Cyberbullying is on the rise, and adverse outcomes related to bullying may include school avoidance, poor academic performance, somatic complaints such as poor appetite and headaches, and increased mental health problems, including depression, suicidal ideation, and attempted suicide (McDougall & Vaillancourt, 2015).

Prevention of bullying behaviors is key. Providers, parents, and school officials must collaborate to teach children to identify bullying and stand up to it safely. Adults must respond quickly and consistently to bullying behavior. Goals include building a safe school environment and creating a community-wide bullying prevention strategy (Stopbullying.gov, n.d.).

Attention Deficit Hyperactivity Disorder

Attention deficit hyperactivity disorder is one of the most commonly diagnosed psychiatric disorders in children, and management has become increasingly complex as new therapies are introduced. It has been reported that pharmacological (e.g., stimulants, nonstimulants, antidepressants, and antipsychotics), psychological (e.g., behavioral, cognitive training, and neurofeedback), and complementary/alternative medicine interventions (e.g., dietary therapy, minerals, herbal therapy, homeopathy, and physical activity) have been found effective in management (Catala-Lopez et al., 2017). Overall, behavioral therapy (an intervention directed at changing behaviors, e.g., problem-solving strategies and social skills training) in combination with stimulants was superior to nonstimulants or stimulant therapy alone, and the most efficacious pharmacological treatments were associated with side effects such as anorexia, weight loss, and insomnia (Catala-Lopez et al., 2017). Due to the importance of and complexity of assessment and management options available, management planning must involve inputs from caregivers, teachers, and specialty providers, such as neurology, psychiatry, and other experts in child development.

Childhood Obesity

Childhood obesity is, perhaps, one of the greatest challenges in our healthcare system. Overweight and obese children are at risk for type 2 diabetes, cardiovascular disease, and psychosocial problems, and obesity during childhood is a strong predictor for obesity in adulthood (Campbell, 2016). Other conditions such as metabolic syndrome, depression, low self-esteem, high cholesterol, asthma, sleep disorders, and nonalcoholic fatty liver disease may result in obese pediatric patients (Mayo Clinic, n.d.). Lifestyle, genetic, and/or hormonal factors may play a role in childhood obesity.

Assessment should include a thorough history of diet including high-calorie foods and sugary drinks, activity levels, family factors, such as an environment where high-calorie foods are always available, psychological factors, such as personal, parental, and family stress, and socioeconomic factors, such as limited access to healthy food or lack of a safe place to exercise (Mayo Clinic, n.d.). Physical examination must focus on vital signs and anthropometric measures and include assessment for conditions such as dental caries, tonsillar hypertrophy, gynecomastia, hepatomegaly, hirsutism, acne, striae, and cervicodorsal hump, among others (Armstrong et al., 2016). Timely referral to supportive services such as nutritional counseling and/or endocrinology is the key management principle, although it is often the primary care provider who plays a key role in educating on the risks of childhood obesity and healthy lifestyle practices. Removal of electronic devices from the bedroom and rules/limits on screen time may be associated with a reduction in childhood obesity (Jong, et al. 2011). Resources to tackle childhood obesity can be found at American Academy of Pediatrics (n.d.).

CARE OF ADOLESCENTS IN PRIMARY CARE SETTINGS

Adolescent patients present to the primary care provider with a set of unique management challenges. Although they may present with many of the acute, episodic, and chronic conditions previously presented, adolescents begin to face an array of conditions more typically found in adult populations. Development is a critical element of adolescent assessment, and issues such as mental health, sexuality, and substance abuse are key areas to include.

Mental Health in the Adolescent Patient

Evidence on the rise of mental health conditions in the adolescent patient is startling. It has been reported that 29% of high school-aged children feel sad and hopeless nearly every day. Furthermore, 16%

reported seriously considering suicide, 13% developed a suicide plan, and 8% tried to commit suicide (Jonovich & Alpert-Gillis, 2014). Therefore, it is imperative that the primary care provider employ strategies to appropriately screen for mental health issues and intervene promptly. One example of an easy-to-use, quick, self-report tool can be found at Bright Futures (n.d.).

Management plans may, of course, involve an antidepressant. Antidepressant therapies work best in combination with psychotherapy, where the adolescent can learn coping skills to deal with psychosocial stressors. However, some recent evidence suggests no clear benefit of treatment with antidepressants for children and adolescents (Oberlander & Miller, 2011). The Food and Drug Administration has also issued a "black box" warning for all antidepressants in young people up to the age of 24 years because of the risk that the drugs might increase suicidal thinking (Cipriani et al., 2016). A significant gap exists between the prevalence of mental health concerns and patients receiving appropriate mental health services (Jonovich & Alpert-Gillis, 2014) so that primary care providers must play a pivotal role in preliminary diagnosis and management.

Adolescent Sexuality and Substance Abuse

Adolescence is a time for experimentation. Primary care office visits provide opportunities for education and healthcare services to prevent sexually transmitted infections, unintended pregnancy, and substance abuse. The American Academy of Pediatrics recommends confidential time during health maintenance visits to discuss sexuality, sexual health promotion, and risk reduction. Additionally, LGBTQ youth may need multiple visits before they disclose their identity; making the office LGBTQ friendly is critical so that the provider is seen as a safe and sympathetic person to whom the adolescent can feel comfortable making sensitive disclosures (Marcell & Burstein, 2017).

In 2019, the National Institute on Drug Abuse (NIDA) launched two screening options on adolescent substance use (NIDA, 2019). As a result, the provider can determine no reported use, low risk, and high risk and intervene accordingly. Introducing screening into practice can normalize discussions, reinforce and promote healthy behaviors, identify those at high risk, and guide interventions and referrals (NIDA, 2019).

Vaping is a current public health crisis that threatens adolescent health. There is an alarming rise in the number of adolescents who have reported vaping behaviors (28%–37% from 2017 to 2018). Adolescents are attracted to the marketing of this technology. It is urgent that they understand the effects of vaping on overall health, the development of the adolescent brain, and the potential for addiction (National Institutes of Health, n.d.). Although the collection and analysis of the evidence is underway, some preliminary known risks of adolescent vaping include the high levels of nicotine found in the products, increased risk of addiction to the adolescent brain, impact on the ability to focus, significant increase in levels of carcinogenic compounds, lung illness, damage to immune system cells, and increase in heart rate and blood pressure resulting in circulatory problems (Martinelli, n.d.). Therefore, screening and intervention are crucial elements of the adolescent well visit.

Fast Facts

- Breastfed infants have a 12% to 24% reduction in the future risk of being overweight or obese.
- Infants must be placed on their backs to sleep until the age of 1 year on a flat, firm surface, which is free from sleep positioners, bumpers, loose bedding, and toys.
- Caregivers need guidance in recognizing the physiological, cognitive, and verbal signs of toilet training readiness and should support children at the appropriate time using effective strategies for success.
- Consistent limits must be placed on screen time ensuring that media does not take the place of adequate sleep, physical activity, and other healthy lifestyle behaviors.
- Cyberbullying is on the rise.
- Approximately one in five children meet the criteria for a mental health disorder.
- Vaping is a current public health crisis that threatens adolescent health.

SUMMARY

This journey through the subspecialties continued with a variety of collaborative clinical practice sessions with physician specialists and NPs practicing in specialty settings. Pediatric and adolescent patients presented with common complaints that often begin with their visit to the primary care provider. This clinical immersion experience led to the identification of hot topics that the primary/urgent care NP is expected to diagnose or perhaps initiate management of in pediatric settings. As always, effective management plans can only be developed once the provider has identified the correct etiology.

References

American Academy of Pediatrics. (2016). *American Academy of Pediatrics announces new recommendations for children's media use.* Retrieved from https://www.aap.org/en-us/about-the-aap/aap-press-room/Pages/American-Academy-of-Pediatrics-Announces-New-Recommendations-for-Childrens-Media-Use.aspx

American Academy of Pediatrics. (n.d.). Retrieved from https://ihcw.aap.org/Pages/default.aspx

American Family Physician. (2017). *SIDS and safe sleeping environments for infants: AAP updates recommendations.* Retrieved from https://www.aafp.org/afp/2017/0615/p806.html

Armstrong, S., Lazorick, S., Hampl, S., Skelton, J. A., Wood, C., Collier, D., & Perrin, E. M. (2016). Physical examination findings among children and adolescents with obesity: An evidence-based review. *Pediatrics, 137*(2), e20151766. Retrieved from https://pediatrics.aappublications.org/content/137/2/e20151766

Bostic, J., & Cullins, L. (2019). *Early identification of mental health problems saves lives.* AAP DC Chapter. Retrieved from http://aapdc.org/early-identification-of-mental-health-problems-saves-lives/

Bright Futures. (n.d.). *Pediatric symptom checklist.* Retrieved from https://www.brightfutures.org/mentalhealth/pdf/professionals/ped_sympton_chklst.pdf

Campbell, K. (2016). Biological, environmental, and social influences on childhood obesity. *Pediatric Research, 79*(1), 205–211.

Catala-Lopez, F., Hutton, B., Nunez-Beltran, A., Page, M., Ridao, M., Macias, D., & Moher, D. (2017). The pharmacological and non-pharmacological treatment of attention deficit hyperactivity disorder in children and adolescents: A systematic review with network meta-analyses of randomized trials. *PLoS One, 12*(7), e0180355. doi:10.1371/journal.pone.0180355

Cipriani, A., Furukawa, T. A., Salanti, G., Chaimani, A., Atkinson, L. Z., Ogawa, Y., &Geddes, J. R. (2016). Comparative efficacy and tolerability of antidepressants for major depressive disorder in children and adolescents: A network meta-analysis. *The Lancet, 388*(10047), 881–890. doi:10.1016/S0140-6736(17)32802-7

Hao, Q., Dong, B., & Wu, T. (2015). Probiotics for preventing acute upper respiratory tract infections. *Cochrane Systematic Review-Intervention.* doi:10.1002/14651858.CD006895.pub3

Hymel, S., & Swearer, S. (2015). Four decades of research on school bullying: An introduction. *American Psychologist, 70*(4), 293–299. doi:10.1037/a0038928

Jonovich, S., & Alpert-Gillis, L. (2014). Impact of pediatric mental health screening on clinical discussion and referral for services. *Clinical Pediatrics, 4*, 364–371. doi:10.1177/0009922813511146

La Leche League International. (n.d.). *Breastfeeding info A to Z.* Retrieved from https://www.llli.org/breastfeeding-info/

Marcell, A. V., & Burstein, G. R. (2017). Sexual and reproductive health care services in the pediatric setting. *Pediatrics, 140*(5), e20172858. Retrieved from https://pediatrics.aappublications.org/content/140/5/e20172858

March of Dimes. (2019). *Safe sleep for your baby*. Retrieved from https://www.marchofdimes.org/baby/safe-sleep-for-your-baby.aspx

Martinelli, K. (n.d.). *Teen vaping: What you need to know*. Retrieved from https://childmind.org/article/teen-vaping-what-you-need-to-know/

Mayo Clinic. (n.d.). *Childhood obesity*. Retrieved from https://www.mayoclinic.org/diseases-conditions/childhood-obesity/symptoms-causes/syc-20354827

McDougall, P., & Vaillancourt, T. (2015). Long-term adult outcomes of peer victimization in childhood and adolescence pathways to adjustment and maladjustment. *American Psychologist, 70*(4), 300–310. doi:10.1037/a0039174

National Institute on Drug Abuse. (2019). *NIDA launches two brief online validated adolescent substance use screening tools*. Retrieved from https://www.drugabuse.gov/nidamed-medical-health-professionals/screening-tools-resources/screening-tools-for-adolescent-substance-use

National Institutes of Health. (n.d.). *Vaping rises among teens*. Retrieved from https://newsinhealth.nih.gov/2019/02/vaping-rises-among-teens

Oberlander, T., & Miller, A. (2011). Antidepressant use in children and adolescents: Practice touch points to guide paediatricians. *Paediatric Child Health, 16*(9), 549–553. doi:10.1093/pch/16.9.549

Oken, E., Fields, D., Lovelady, C., & Redman, L. (2017). TOS scientific position statement: Breastfeeding and obesity. *Obesity, 25*(11), 1864–1866. doi:10.1002/oby.22024

Stopbullying.gov. (n.d.). *Stop bullying on the spot*. Retrieved from www.stopbullying.gov

Sung, V., Collett, S., de Gooyer, T., Hickcock, H., Tang, M., & Wake, M. (2013). Probiotics to prevent or treat excessive infant crying: A systemic review and meta-analysis. *JAMA Pediatrics, 167*(12), 1150–1157. doi:10.1001/jamapediatrics.2013.2572

Wolraich, M. (2016). *American Academy of Pediatrics guide to toilet trailing* (2nd ed.). New York, NY: Bantam Books.

17

Practice Essentials for Psychiatry

The adult client will often present to the primary care setting with mental health symptoms. Although some may be appropriate for the primary care provider to diagnose and manage, many conditions may be persistent or significant enough to be referred to the mental health specialist for evaluation and management. The seasoned practitioner is knowledgeable on the standards of care for the client with a psychiatric condition, particularly the red flags to assess and refer for a consultation with a psychiatrist. However, delays in mental health treatment may occur. Evidence suggests that a collaborative care model, where the client's physical and mental health needs are addressed in one setting, results in positive outcomes. Here, tools such as symptom rating scales and clinical decision-making algorithms can be used effectively by the primary care provider to identify the client's mental healthcare needs and refer accordingly (McKnight, 2016).

It is likely that the majority of clients seen in the primary care setting have a clinical problem with a significant psychological or behavioral component. The management of these clients' healthcare needs can challenge provider time and resources.

Fast Facts

Strategies for fostering a stronger client–provider relationship include being present, using physical touch when appropriate and open body language (turning away from computer), employing active listening and reflection, instilling hope and power, and expressing empathy (Sherman, Miller, Keuler, Trump, & Mandrich, 2017).

Sherman et al. (2017) provide practical examples for management such as encouraging the patient to draw on social supports, increasing the frequency of visits, assisting in focusing on gratitude, teaching breathing and mindfulness exercises, prescribing physical exercise, and encouraging the creation of a routine or schedule.

DEPRESSION

Clients will typically first report depressive symptoms to the primary care provider. The American Psychiatric Association's *Diagnostic and Statistical Manual of Mental Disorders*, Fifth Edition, defines a client with major depressive disorder as having either depressed mood or markedly diminished pleasure in most activities for most days for at least 2 weeks, coupled with at least four of the following: appetite disturbance, sleep disturbance, motor retardation or agitation, lack of energy, feelings of worthlessness or excessive guilt, decreased concentration, and/or recurrent thoughts of death or suicide (Koirala & Anand, 2018). The client with suicidal thoughts or a history of suicide attempts should receive an immediate psychological evaluation/risk assessment by a psychiatrist or trained mental health specialist.

As psychotherapy has been shown to be as effective as antidepressants for mild-to-moderate major depression, a referral to a therapist should be considered. Other nonpharmacologic strategies to assist the client in the management of depressive symptoms involve managing stressors, engaging social and community support, dealing with stigma and discrimination, and managing comorbidities (Ng, How, & Ng, 2017). If pharmacologic management of depressive symptoms is also indicated, antidepressants should be initiated at the starting dose and then gradually increased until a therapeutic response is achieved, and clients should be educated on the anticipated time frame needed to assess for efficacy. Categories of antidepressants with select agents and recommended starting doses are provided in Table 17.1 (Ng et al., 2017).

Table 17.1

Antidepressants		
Selective serotonin reuptake inhibitors	Citalopram 20 mg	Fluvoxamine CR 100 mg
	Escitalopram 10 mg	Paroxetine 20 mg
	Fluoxetine 20 mg	Paroxetine CR 25 mg
	Fluvoxamine 50 mg	Sertraline 50 mg

(continued)

Table 17.1

Antidepressants (*continued*)

Serotonin–norepinephrine reuptake inhibitors	Desvenlafaxine 25–50 mg Duloxetine 30–60 mg Levomilnacipran 20 mg	Milnacipran 12.5 mg Venlafaxine 37.5–75 mg Venlafaxine XR 37.5–75 mg
Atypicals	Bupropion 200 mg Mirtazapine 15 mg Bupropion hydrobromide 24 hr, 174 mg	Bupropion SR 12 hr, 150 mg Bupropion XL 24 hr, 150 mg
Serotonin modulators	Nefazodone 200 mg Trazodone 100 mg	Vilazodone 10 mg Vortioxetine 10 mg
Tricyclics	Amitriptyline 25 mg Amoxapine 25 mg Clomipramine 25 mg Desipramine 25 mg Doxepin 25 mg	Imipramine 25 mg Maprotiline 25 mg Nortriptyline 25 mg Protriptyline 10 mg Trimipramine 25 mg
Monoamine oxidase inhibitors	Isocarboxazid 10 mg Selegiline transdermal 6 mg/24 hr patch	Tranylcypromine 10 mg Phenelzine 15 mg

Source: Data from Ng, C., How, C., & Ng, Y. (2017). Managing depression in primary care. *Singapore Medical Journal, 58*(8), 459–466. doi:10.11622/smedj.2017080

Not all pharmacologic agents are appropriate for all clients, nor are all antidepressants appropriate to initiate in all healthcare settings. It is critical that the provider is knowledgeable on appropriate first-line agents, conducts a thorough assessment of the client's symptoms and comorbid condition, severity of depressive symptoms, and overall mental health risk prior to and during the pharmacologic management of a major depressive disorder, and consults with a psychiatrist when indicated.

BIPOLAR DISORDER

In addition to the previously described symptoms of major depressive disorder, the client may also report manic symptoms, or the presence of persistently elevated, expansive, or irritable mood with increased activity for >1 week, as well as at least three of the following: impaired functioning (four features are required if mood is only irritable), inflated self-esteem or grandiosity, decreased need for sleep, pressured speech, racing thoughts, distractibility, and/or excessive involvement in pleasurable, high-risk activities (Koirala & Anand, 2018). Although the seasoned clinician is aware that the client with bipolar disorder is most often treated with mood stabilizers, antidepressants, or neuroleptic drugs, it is likely most appropriate for the client with mania to be managed primarily by a mental health specialist. It is, however, critical that the primary care provider understand that some medications can induce manic symptoms. Examples include select antidepressants, stimulants, steroids, antiparkinsonian or dopaminergic drugs, levothyroxine, cyclosporine, antibiotics such as ciprofloxacin or gentamicin, chloroquine, or some cancer drugs such as fluorouracil or ifosfamide (Koirala & Anand, 2018). In addition, there are some conditions associated with bipolar disorders to understand and assess for. For instance, migraines, thyroid disease, obesity, diabetes, hypertension, cardiovascular disease, chronic obstructive pulmonary disease, HIV, hepatitis C, sexually transmitted infections, substance abuse, and accidents/injuries (Koirala & Anand, 2018). As always, a team approach among psychiatrist and/or psychiatric nurse practitioner, primary care provider, therapist/social worker, and other members of the interdisciplinary team will result in optimal healthcare outcomes for the client with bipolar disorder.

ANXIETY

Generalized anxiety disorder is one of the most common mental health conditions reported to the primary care provider. Excessive and persistent worrying that occurs on more days than not for at least 6 months is the hallmark feature, yet clients may also present with symptoms of restlessness, irritability, apprehensiveness, poor sleep, fatigue, difficulty relaxing, poor concentration, headaches, neck pain, shoulder pain, and back pain. Possible physical causes of anxiety symptoms should be excluded, such as hyperthyroidism, so a workup including a complete blood count, chemistry panel, serum thyrotropin, urinalysis, electrocardiogram, and urine or serum toxicology analysis for drugs or medications should be performed (Baldwin, 2019). Cognitive behavioral therapy and applied relaxation have been found to be effective, and medications including selective serotonin reuptake inhibitors and serotonin–norepinephrine reuptake inhibitors as listed earlier may be considered if nonpharmacologic modalities have not demonstrated improved outcomes.

Fast Facts

Benzodiazepines have been found to be efficacious in the treatment of generalized anxiety disorder; however, concerns about risks of dependence and tolerance have contributed to a decline in their use (Bystritsky, 2019). Other therapies such as buspirone, pregabalin, other antidepressants, atypical antipsychotics, anticonvulsants, and hydroxyzine have demonstrated efficacy in managing symptoms of generalized anxiety disorder.

The skillful practitioner is aware that the client with generalized anxiety disorder typically presents with increased rates of depression, substance abuse, posttraumatic stress disorder, obsessive–compulsive disorder, and medically unexplained chronic pain, so assessment for comorbid conditions is critical (Baldwin, 2019). As increased cardiovascular health may be associated with this condition, screening and management are integral roles of the primary care provider.

EATING DISORDERS

Eating disorders such as anorexia nervosa, bulimia nervosa, and binge eating disorder most commonly affect white adolescent girls and young women but can affect clients of all ages and backgrounds. The primary care provider plays a key role in screening for these disorders. Once identified, a comprehensive management program involves a team approach consisting of psychiatry and other mental health experts, the primary care provider, and a nutritionist who all play key roles in treatment (Yager, 2019). Early diagnosis and intervention are associated with improved outcomes (Sangvai, 2016). The assessment for and management of complications of eating disorders may be appropriate roles of the primary care provider. More significant conditions may involve inpatient management and therapies, which are beyond the scope and breadth of the primary care setting.

SUBSTANCE USE DISORDERS

Although most individuals with addiction do not receive treatment, screening for substance use disorders and referral when indicated are important roles of the primary care provider (Saitz & Daaleman, 2017).

Most primary care providers incorporate inquiry regarding smoking habits, alcohol intake, and illicit drug use. More recently, the client's health history explores vaping habits and the improper use of opioids. Time is a challenge in most primary care settings. Furthermore, providers may lack the knowledge, experience, or confidence in the management of substance use disorders (Saitz & Daaleman, 2017).

All primary care providers should demonstrate competency in guiding the client through the process of smoking cessation. The 5 A's model encourages the clinician to *ask* patients about smoking, *advise* all smokers to quit, *assess* their readiness to quit, *assist* them with their smoking cessation effort, and *arrange* for follow-up visits or contact (Park, 2019). The first-line pharmacologic management for smoking cessation in the general population includes nicotine replacement therapy, varenicline, and bupropion (Rigotti, 2019). Park (2019) reports that other nonpharmacologic measures that have demonstrated efficacy to support the client in smoking cessation include individual, group, telephone counseling, text messaging, web resources, and use of phone apps.

Fast Facts

- Strategies for fostering a stronger client–provider relationship include being present, using physical touch when appropriate and open body language (turning away from computer), employing active listening and reflection, instilling hope and power, and expressing empathy.
- A client with major depressive disorder has either depressed mood or markedly diminished pleasure in most activities for most days for at least 2 weeks, coupled with appetite disturbance, sleep disturbance, motor retardation or agitation, lack of energy, feelings of worthlessness or excessive guilt, decreased concentration, and/or recurrent thoughts of death or suicide.
- The client with suicidal thoughts or a history of suicide attempts should receive an immediate psychological evaluation/risk assessment by a psychiatrist or trained mental health specialist.
- Excessive and persistent worrying that occurs on more days than not for at least 6 months is the hallmark feature of generalized anxiety disorder, yet clients may also present with symptoms of restlessness, irritability, apprehensiveness, poor sleep, fatigue, difficulty relaxing, poor concentration, headaches, neck pain, shoulder pain, and back pain.
- Early diagnosis and treatment are associated with improved eating disorder outcomes.

(continued)

(continued)

- The first-line pharmacologic management for smoking cessation in the general population includes nicotine replacement therapy, varenicline, and bupropion.

SUMMARY

This journey through the subspecialties continued with a collaborative clinical practice session with physician specialists and nurse practitioners practicing in specialty settings. Clients presented with common mental health complaints often begin with their visit to the primary care provider. This clinical immersion experience led to the identification of psychiatric conditions that the primary care provider is expected to diagnose or perhaps initiate management of. A mental health specialist may be consulted for emergent psychiatric conditions. As always, effective management plans can only be developed once the provider has identified the correct etiology.

References

Baldwin, D. (2019). *Generalized anxiety disorder in adults: Epidemiology, pathogenesis, clinical manifestations, course, assessment, and diagnosis.* UpToDate. Retrieved from https://www.uptodate.com/contents/generalized-anxiety-disorder-in-adults-epidemiology-pathogenesis-clinical-manifestations-course-assessment-and-diagnosis

Bystritsky, A. (2019). *Pharmacotherapy for generalized anxiety disorder in adults.* UpToDate. Retrieved from https://www.uptodate.com/contents/pharmacotherapy-for-generalized-anxiety-disorder-in-adults

Koirala, P., & Anand, A. (2018). Diagnosing and treating bipolar disorder in primary care. *Cleveland Clinic Journal of Medicine, 85*(8), 601–608. doi:10.3949/ccjm.85gr.18003

McKnight, W. (2016). Primary care's rising role in behavioral health requires specialty partnerships. *Clinical Psychiatry News.* Retrieved from https://www.mdedge.com/psychiatry/article/111689/mental-health/primary-cares-rising-role-behavioral-health-requires

Ng, C., How, C., & Ng, Y. (2017). Managing depression in primary care. *Singapore Medical Journal, 58*(8), 459–466. doi:10.11622/smedj.2017080

Park, E. (2019). *Behavioral approaches to smoking cessation.* UpToDate. Retrieved from https://www.uptodate.com/contents/behavioral-approaches-to-smoking-cessation

Rigotti, N. (2019). *Pharmacotherapy for smoking cessation in adults.* UpToDate. Retrieved from https://www.uptodate.com/contents/pharmacotherapy-for-smoking-cessation-in-adults

Saitz, R., & Daaleman, T. P. (2017). Now is the time to address substance use disorders in primary care. *Annals of Family Medicine, 15*(4), 306–308. doi:10.1370/afm.2111

Sangvai, D. (2016). Eating disorders in the primary care setting. *Prim Care,* *43*(2), 301–312. doi:10.1016/j.pop.2016.01.007

Sherman, M., Miller, L., Keuler, M., Trump, L., & Mandrich, M. (2017). Managing behavioral health issues in primary care: 6 five-minute tools. *Family Practice Management, 24*(2), 31–35.

Yager, J. (2019). *Eating disorders: Overview of epidemiology, clinical features, and diagnosis.* UpToDate. Retrieved from https://www.uptodate.com/contents/eating-disorders-overview-of-epidemiology-clinical-features-and-diagnosis

18

Practice Essentials for Pulmonology

Clients often seek care in primary care settings for symptoms related to the pulmonary system. At times, this is appropriate, and a diagnosis can be made and symptoms managed with optimal outcomes achieved. More severe, persistent, or difficult-to-control conditions may often require a referral to a specialist or emergency services to formulate a diagnosis and initiate a management plan.

OBSTRUCTIVE SLEEP APNEA

Adult and older adult clients commonly report symptoms of poor sleep, daytime fatigue, difficulty concentrating, observed episodes of stopped breathing during sleep, awakening with dry mouth or sore throat, morning headaches, nighttime sweating, decreased libido, and/or loud snoring to their primary care provider. Snoring, obesity, advancing age, chronic nasal congestion, asthma, family history, and male gender are known risk factors for obstructive sleep apnea; while postmenopausal women are affected by obstructive sleep apnea equally, as are those with type 2 diabetes, resistant hypertension, or ischemic heart disease (Chai-Coetzer, Antic, & McEnvoy, 2015). Clients who report these symptoms are deemed at risk and are generally referred to a sleep specialist for consultation or directly for polysomnography, or a sleep study, by the primary care provider.

If a diagnosis of obstructive sleep apnea is made as a result, lifestyle changes (see Box 18.1) and treatment options such as a continuous positive airway pressure equipment, a mouthpiece, or surgery may be indicated. Potential complications of obstructive sleep apnea

BOX 18.1   RECOMMENDED LIFESTYLE CHANGES FOR CLIENTS WITH OBSTRUCTIVE SLEEP APNEA

- Weight loss
- Regular exercise
- Moderate intake of alcohol, if at all, and refrain several hours before bedtime
- Smoking cessation
- Nasal decongestants
- Antihistamines
- Avoidance of at-risk sleeping positions, such as sleeping on the back
- Avoidance of sedative medications, such as antianxiety drugs or sleeping pills

Source: Data from Mayo Clinic. (2019b, June 5). *Obstructive sleep apnea: Overview*. Retrieved from https://www.mayoclinic.org/diseases-conditions/obstructive-sleep-apnea/symptoms-causes/syc-20352090

include daytime fatigue, cardiovascular disease/arrhythmias, glaucoma, complications with medications, general anesthesia, or surgery, and/or relationship problems (Mayo Clinic, 2019a).

Overall, a collaborative approach to management between the client and family with the primary care provider in concert with the pulmonary specialist and/or a sleep specialist, which includes a number of lifestyle changes coupled with one or more of the modalities described earlier, will foster improved healthcare outcomes for the adult client who presents with obstructive sleep apnea.

COUGH

Clients commonly present to primary care settings complaining of a cough. The cough may be acute or chronic, frequent or intermittent, or occur in isolation or along with a number of other accompanying symptoms. It is critical that the primary care provider determine the correct etiology of the cough in order to formulate and implement an effective management plan. The seasoned provider is well aware that a cough can be related to a pulmonary condition, as well as a disorder of other body systems, such as the gastrointestinal or cardiovascular systems. The management of a cough that is triggered by asthma is presented in Chapter 3, Practice Essentials for Allergy and Immunology.

Bronchitis

When the client presents with an acute cough; with or without sputum production, fever, nasal congestion, dyspnea, chest pain while coughing, or headache; and signs of lower respiratory tract infection in the absence of another condition, such as chronic obstructive pulmonary disease (COPD), pneumonia, or sinusitis, a diagnosis of acute bronchitis is made. The physical examination may reveal a wheeze and rhonchi that typically improve with cough. Laboratory testing is not indicated for evaluation, and imaging is only used to rule out pneumonia such as in the client with abnormal vital signs (e.g., tachypnea, tachycardia), in the client with abnormal lung examination findings, and/or in the client older than 75 years (Kinkade & Long, 2016).

The skillful practitioner is aware that the presence of a fever >100°F indicates probing further for the presence of influenza or pneumonia, and sputum production does not correlate with bacterial infection. Clients should be clearly educated that the duration of cough may be 2 to 3 weeks, and antibiotic therapy is not indicated for uncomplicated acute bronchitis to the otherwise healthy adult client. Evidence-based treatment options include recommending dextromethorphan, guaifenesin, or honey to manage symptoms and avoiding β2-agonists unless wheezing is present (Kinkade & Long, 2016).

Community-Acquired Pneumonia

The presence of an acute infection of the pulmonary parenchyma acquired outside of the hospital indicates community-acquired pneumonia; the risk increases with recent viral respiratory tract infection, such as influenza, advancing age (>65 years), recent anesthesia, drug/alcohol use, smoking, crowded living conditions, residence in low-income settings, exposure to environmental toxins, and chronic comorbidities, such as COPD, asthma, congestive heart failure, stroke, seizure, diabetes, malnutrition, dysphagia, and immunocompromised status (Ramirez, 2019). The typical clinical presentation includes fever/chills, cough (with or without sputum production), pleuritic chest pain, malaise, anorexia, and dyspnea. The quality of the respiratory distress may differ significantly. Adventitious breath sounds may include rales/crackles and rhonchi. Tachycardia, leukocytosis, and/or hypoxia may also be present, and older clients may present with subtle mental status changes. An infiltrate is detected on the chest radiograph. There is no direct evidence to suggest that CT scanning improves outcomes, and cost is so high hat routine CT scans are not recommended (Ramirez, 2019).

Most clients with community-acquired pneumonia can be managed outside of the acute care setting. Ramirez (2019) reports that empirical management includes amoxicillin plus a macrolide or doxycycline as a first-line treatment; amoxicillin–clavulanate is recommended for clients with major comorbidities, smokers, or those who have used antibiotics within the past 3 months; and fluoroquinolones are indicated in those who cannot tolerate the earlier therapies or those with a history of structural lung disease. Older clients, those who are cognitively impaired or who demonstrate potential issues with oral medication adherence, or those with hypoxia should be evaluated for hospitalization. Finally, follow-up imaging is not indicated in clients whose symptoms resolve following treatment.

Influenza

Primary care practitioners play an important role in the prevention, diagnosis, and management of the client with influenza. Although most strains of seasonal influenza are self-limiting, influenza is a severe acute viral respiratory illness that can cause significant mortality in the elderly client, as well as in other at-risk populations (Hart, 2015). Although there are a variety of variants of the influenza virus, this section will focus on the care of the adult client who presents following exposure to seasonal influenza.

Fast Facts

Pneumonia is the most common complication of influenza. Hart (2015) reports that American Indians/Alaska Natives, those with morbid obesity (body mass index ≥ 40), pregnant or postpartum women, clients who receive long-term aspirin therapy, adults over 65 years of age or who reside in long-term care facilities, and clients who are immunocompromised or present with chronic pulmonary (e.g., asthma), cardiovascular (except hypertension alone), renal, hepatic, hematologic (e.g., sickle cell disease), and metabolic disorders (e.g., diabetes mellitus) or neurologic and neurodevelopment conditions (e.g., cerebral palsy, epilepsy, stroke, intellectual disability, moderate-to-severe developmental delay, muscular dystrophy, or spinal cord injury) are at higher risk for complications resulting from seasonal influenza.

The client with seasonal influenza will typically present with a sudden onset of fever, headache, myalgia, and fatigue accompanied by cough, sore throat, and nasal discharge. Evidence suggests that the majority of clients with uncomplicated influenza experience symptoms for 3 to 7 days and will clear the virus after 5 to 10 days of symptom onset with no treatment (Hart, 2015).

Influenza vaccination is an important measure in the protection against influenza and, so, education on vaccination is a paramount role of the primary care provider. Diagnosis in outpatient settings is made based on clinical symptomatology and assessment, as well as with the use of rapid influenza diagnosis testing, which is 90% to 95% specific and 50% to 70% sensitive (Hart, 2015). The goal of influenza management is support and symptom management using over-the-counter fever, pain, and cough medications. Early (within 48 hours of illness onset) antiviral treatment can shorten the duration of fever and illness symptoms and may reduce the risk of complications from influenza. The avoidance of complication and the need for hospitalization are of paramount concern. Currently available antiviral medications include oseltamivir (Tamiflu), zanamivir (Relenza), peramivir (Rapivab), or baloxavir (Xofluza; Mayo Clinic, 2019c). Providers should remain current by routinely reviewing the Centers for Disease Control and Prevention's (2020) "FluView Interactive" website for the latest information regarding influenza strains and antiviral resistance.

Chronic Obstructive Pulmonary Disease

Although the client with COPD typically requires consultation with a specialty provider, it is typically the primary care provider who is responsible for the prevention of complication and management of individual symptoms, such as dyspnea, productive cough, fatigue, and limited exercise tolerance. Improved outcomes include the client's adherence to the plan of care, the reduction of symptoms, and improved quality of life (Sethi, 2018).

Diagnosis must be differentiated from asthma and should not be made on spirometry alone. Sethi (2018) describes how spirometry results are used in concert with a thorough history, and focused physical examination considering client age, onset, progression of symptoms, and social/occupational risk is the hallmark of COPD diagnosis. The hallmark of management of COPD involves inhaled bronchodilators. Primary care practice must involve the assessment for appropriate mode of delivery and include training on proper use. An effective management plan incorporates a focus on the reduction of exacerbation and minimizes (if not avoids) hospitalization. Oral glucocorticoids may be effective during an exacerbation, and careful monitoring of adverse effects is indicated. The difficult-to-manage clients (those with frequent exacerbation and need for hospitalization) should most likely receive care provided by a pulmonologist (Sethi, 2018). According to Sethi (2018), best practices include encouraging smoking cessation and healthy lifestyle behaviors, providing routine patient monitoring, assessing ongoing treatment goals, and monitoring medication adherence.

LUNG CANCER SCREENING

Annual low-dose CAT scan screening is recommended for lung cancer in certain high-risk individuals. The seasoned primary care provider is aware that the adult clients aged 55 to 80 years who have a 30-pack-year smoking history and currently smoke or have quit within the past 15 years are at high risk for the development of lung cancer. Furthermore, the primary care provider should consider the initiation of annual screening starting at age 50 to 79 years in clients with a 20-pack-year smoking history and additional comorbid conditions that produce a cumulative risk for cancer (Kwoh, Kaneshiro, Paige, & Betancourt, 2018).

Kwoh et al. (2018) report that the primary care provider is often challenged by decisions regarding which nodules may represent early lung cancer and therefore need follow-up imaging. The primary care provider should be primarily responsible for initiating discussion with patients about lung cancer screening, implementing lung cancer screening, and managing follow-up. As not having enough time to address lung cancer screening may be a barrier to screening, a referral to a specialty provider is most often appropriate (Triplette et al., 2018).

Fast Facts

- Snoring, obesity, advancing age, chronic nasal congestion, asthma, family history, and male gender are known risk factors for obstructive sleep apnea; postmenopausal women are affected by obstructive sleep apnea equally, as are those with type 2 diabetes, resistant hypertension, or ischemic heart disease.
- Clients should be clearly educated that the duration of cough may be 2 to 3 weeks, and antibiotic therapy is not indicated for uncomplicated acute bronchitis to the otherwise healthy adult client.

(continued)

(continued)

■ The empirical management of community-acquired pneumonia includes amoxicillin plus a macrolide or doxycycline as a first-line treatment; amoxicillin–clavulanate is recommended for clients with major comorbidities, smokers, or those who have used antibiotics within the past 3 months; and fluoroquinolones are indicated in those who cannot tolerate the earlier therapies or those with a history of structural lung disease.

■ The majority of clients with uncomplicated influenza experience symptoms for 3 to 7 days and will clear the virus after 5 to 10 days of symptom onset with no treatment.

■ The best practices in COPD management include encouraging smoking cessation and healthy lifestyle behaviors, providing routine patient monitoring, assessing ongoing treatment goals, and monitoring medication adherence.

■ Annual low-dose CAT scan screening is recommended for lung cancer in certain high-risk individuals.

SUMMARY

This journey through the subspecialties continued with a collaborative clinical practice session with physician specialists and nurse practitioners practicing in specialty settings. Clients presented with common complaints of the pulmonary system that often begin with their visit to the primary care provider. This clinical immersion experience led to the identification of conditions that the primary care provider is expected to diagnose or perhaps refer to a specialist in pulmonology. As always, effective management plans can only be developed once the provider has identified the correct etiology.

References

Centers for Disease Control and Prevention. (2020). *Influenza (Flu)*. Retrieved from https://www.cdc.gov/flu/weekly/index.htm

Chai-Coetzer, C., Antic, N., & McEnvoy, R. (2015). Identifying and managing sleep disorders in primary care. *The Lancet. Respiratory Medicine, 3*(5), 337–339. doi:10.1016/S2213-2600(15)00141-1

Hart, A. (2015). Respecting influenza: An evidence-based overview for primary care nurse practitioners. *The Nurse Practitioner, 11*(1), 41–48. doi:10.1016/j.nurpra.2014.10.023

Kinkade, S., & Long, N. (2016). Acute bronchitis. *American Family Physician, 94*(7), 560–565.

Kwoh, E., Kaneshiro, C., Paige, N., & Betancourt, J. (2018). The top 10 pulmonary pearls for primary care physicians. *Mayo Clinic Proceedings, 93*(8), 1131–1138. Retrieved from https://www.mayoclinicproceedings.org/article/S0025-6196(18)30490-7/pdf

Mayo Clinic. (2019a, June 5). *Obstructive sleep apnea: Diagnosis.* Retrieved from https://www.mayoclinic.org/diseases-conditions/obstructive-sleep-apnea/diagnosis-treatment/drc-20352095

Mayo Clinic. (2019b, June 5). *Obstructive sleep apnea: Overview.* Retrieved from https://www.mayoclinic.org/diseases-conditions/obstructive-sleep-apnea/symptoms-causes/syc-20352090

Mayo Clinic. (2019c, October 4). *Influenza (flu).* Retrieved from https://www.mayoclinic.org/diseases-conditions/flu/diagnosis-treatment/drc-20351725

Ramirez, J. (2019). *Overview of community-acquired pneumonia in adults.* UpToDate. Retrieved from https://www.uptodate.com/contents/overview-of-community-acquired-pneumonia-in-adults/print

Sethi, S. (2018). *Effective management of COPD in primary care: Challenges and opportunities.* Retrieved from https://www.ajmc.com/contributor/sanjay-sethi/2018/11/effective-management-of-copd-in-primary-care-challenges-and-opportunities

Triplette, M., Kross, E. K., Mann, B. A., Elmore, J. G., Slatore, C. G., Shahrir, S., & Crothers, K. (2018). *An assessment of primary care and pulmonary provider perspectives on lung cancer screening.* Retrieved from https://www.atsjournals.org/doi/pdf/10.1513/AnnalsATS.201705-392OC

19

Practice Essentials for Rheumatology

The adult client may present to the primary care setting with a variety of rheumatologic symptoms. Although many of these are appropriate for the primary care provider to diagnose and manage, some conditions may be persistent or significant enough to be referred to the nephrologist. The skillful provider is knowledgeable on the standards of care for the client with musculoskeletal disease coupled with a variety of systemic autoimmune conditions, as well as the red flags to assess and refer for a consultation with the specialty provider.

RHEUMATOID ARTHRITIS

Clients present to primary care settings complaining of symptoms of polyarthritis, typically affecting the hands and the feet. Often, there is morning stiffness or soreness reported, as well as systemic symptoms such as fatigue, weight loss, and low-grade fever. When these persist for ≥6 weeks, a diagnosis of rheumatoid arthritis should be considered (Goldberg, 2017). Upon physical assessment, the skillful practitioner is sure to assess for observable joint inflammation, which includes redness, warmth, and swelling. When therapy is initiated early , the outcomes are often better. Thus, the primary care provider must collaborate with the rheumatologist in both symptom management and control of comorbid conditions such as cardiovascular disease, depression, sleep disturbances, and osteoporosis (Goldberg, 2017).

Although a referral to a rheumatologist is indicated, a preliminary workup may include an erythrocyte sedimentation rate or C-reactive protein (CRP), as well as a rheumatoid factor or the anti-citrullinated peptide antibody. Furthermore, Goldberg (2017) suggests prednisone

10 to 15 mg daily for early rheumatoid arthritis to control symptoms while the client waits for a consult with the specialty provider.

SYSTEMIC LUPUS ERYTHEMATOSUS

The primary care provider plays a key role in the early identification and evaluation of the symptoms of autoimmune diseases, such as systemic lupus erythematosus, as well as the management of mild, stable diseases, whereas more severe forms of the condition should be managed in collaboration with a specialist. The clinical profile of systemic lupus erythematosus is complex, relapsing and remitting, challenging, and unpredictable, affecting various organ systems (e.g., musculoskeletal, skin, hematologic, renal, neuropsychiatric, cardiovascular, and respiratory systems) with variable degrees of severity. Early recognition, control of exacerbation, and optimization of care are the primary principles of management (Gergianaki & Bertsias, 2018).

Due to the high sensitivity, the antinuclear antibodies (ANAs) test is recommended as an initial lupus screening test. Gergianaki and Bertsias (2018) add that specificity is low for the ANA, as a positive result can be found in other autoimmune diseases, such as autoimmune thyroiditis, autoimmune liver diseases, and myasthenia. In addition, anti–double-strand DNA can be used for both diagnosis and evaluation of disease activity, and anti-Sm antibodies can also be indicated due to their high specificity for lupus.

In general, lupus is managed using glucocorticoids and/or antimalarial drugs, along with immunosuppressive or biologic agents (Gergianaki & Bertsias, 2018). Additional therapies are directed toward symptom management and/or control of system specific(s) targeted by the disease.

Fast Facts

Currently, the same guidelines for cancer screening as the general population are recommended; immunizations against pneumococcus and influenza are given; and live virus vaccines are contraindicated when the client is symptomatic of an exacerbation or receiving immunosuppressive treatments (including prednisone; Gergianaki & Bertsias, 2018).

Additionally, it has been reported that smoking cessation, weight control, and physical exercise are important in this population, especially with those with increased cardiovascular risk. As lupus nephritis and neuropsychiatric lupus are the most significant complications, it is critical that the seasoned primary care provider is certain to evaluate for signs of renal disease, as well as neurologic and psychiatric manifestations such as seizures, cognitive dysfunction, psychosis, or depression. Furthermore, due to the association of thrombosis and pregnancy morbidity, all providers involved in the management of the pregnant client with lupus must be aware of this risk and monitor and refer accordingly (Gergianaki & Bertsias, 2018).

FATIGUE

Although also described in Chapter 11, Practice Essentials for Neurology, the client with a history of conditions such as systemic lupus erythematosus or rheumatoid arthritis may present to the primary care setting. Evidence suggests that some classes of drugs may be effective in treating clients with fatigue, supporting the inflammatory background of the symptoms. Examples include IL-6-blocking agents, tumor necrosis factor-α-blocking agents, and biological disease-modifying antirheumatic drugs (Sanicki & Ozbalkan, 2015). It is likely inappropriate for the primary care practitioner to prescribe these therapies; it is, however, important for them to be familiar with some options and refer the client to the experienced specialty provider in their area to appropriately manage symptoms of chronic fatigue.

Furthermore, these chronically fatigued clients often have reduced exercise capacity, chronic pain, poor sleep patterns, anxiety, and depression. The seasoned provider is certain to assess for comorbid conditions and intervene appropriately. Evidence suggests that serotonin–norepinephrine reuptake inhibitors, selective serotonin reuptake inhibitors, or tricyclic antidepressants could help improve these symptoms, and patient education directed toward the incorporation of cognitive behavioral therapy, activity pacing, energy conservation, increasing physical activity, getting regular exercise, relaxation exercises, rest–activity balance, balanced diet, lifestyle moderation, stress management, time management, and sleep hygiene should be considered to augment pharmacologic management (Sanicki & Ozbalkan, 2015).

SJOGREN'S SYNDROME

Clients who present with dry eyes and dry mouth should be evaluated for Sjogren's syndrome. This chronic autoimmune inflammatory disorder results in diminished lacrimal and salivary gland function. Often, this condition is associated with rheumatoid arthritis and systemic lupus erythematosus (Baer, 2019). The patient's education should include the use of artificial tears and good oral hygiene. As fatigue is another frequently reported symptom, treatment with rituximab should be considered in collaboration with the specialty provider (Sanicki & Ozbalkan, 2015). Smoking cessation, a good diet, and nutrition are other elements of care to be promoted by the primary care provider.

GOUT

Frequently, the client will present to the primary care setting complaining of a painful joint—typically, the ankle, foot, knee, toe, or elbow. If the affected joint is stiff, swollen, tender, red, and/or warm to touch, suspicion should be raised to evaluate for gout. A serum uric acid level should be performed and evaluated to assist in the diagnosis of gout.

Fast Facts

Taking into consideration the patient's preference, renal function, and comorbidities, first-line treatments for the management of an exacerbation of gout include a nonsteroidal anti-inflammatory drug or low-dose colchicine 500 mcg two to four times daily; prednisone can be considered for those who are intolerant of other first-line agents (Mallen, Davenport, Hui, Nuki, & Roddy, 2017). Elevation, rest, and ice should also be recommended for symptom relief.

The client with gout is at increased risk of cardiovascular disease, so screening for and management of hypertension, diabetes mellitus, and dyslipidemia are important components of primary care. In addition, it has been reported that thiazide and loop diuretics should be avoided, as they may cause hyperuricemia (Mallen et al., 2017). The client's education must incorporate avoidance of high-purine foods, sugar-sweetened soft drinks, or excess alcohol intake.

As gout is now considered to be a chronic inflammatory arthritis rather than an acute episodic condition, earlier initiation of urate-lowering therapies to prevent attacks is recommended. Low-dose allopurinol is a first-line therapy. Clients can be started at 50 to 100 mg daily and gradually titrated up at 50 to 100 mg increments every 4 weeks until the target uric acid level has been achieved (maximum 900 mg per day; Mallen et al., 2017). Other treatment options include febuxostat when allopurinol is not tolerated.

SPONDYLOARTHROPATHIES

Ankylosing spondylitis and psoriatic arthritis are examples of spondyloarthropathies that may result in chronic pain and fatigue. Ankylosing spondylitis primarily affects the sacroiliac joints and spine. Typically, this condition is evaluated and managed by a rheumatologist, but the primary care provider may play a collaborative role in symptom management. Evidence suggests that anti-inflammatory drugs are very effective for controlling pain and that regular physical activity is effective in reducing fatigue (Yu & van Tubergen, 2019).

It has been further reported that many of the agents used to treat the symptoms of conditions such as psoriatic arthritis are similar to those used in the management of rheumatoid arthritis or the cutaneous manifestations of psoriasis. Overall, interventions should be aimed at controlling inflammation and preventing discomfort, joint damage, and disability. A specialist should be consulted early in the disease process to promote improved client outcomes, and a collaborative care model that involves rheumatology, dermatology, and primary care providers is encouraged (Gladman & Ritchlin, 2019). Comorbidities such as diabetes, metabolic syndrome, fatty liver, coronary artery disease, depression, and hyperuricemia should be evaluated and managed accordingly. Education on the nonpharmacologic management of symptoms should be provided. For instance, exercise, physical therapy, occupational therapy, stress management, and weight reduction may play an important role in managing psoriatic arthritis (Gladman & Ritchlin, 2019).

SCLERODERMA

Clients with fatigue, joint pain, puffy swollen fingers and/or non-pitting edema of the hands, skin thickening/tightening/ulcerations, abnormal nailfolds, cutaneous hyperpigmentation, calcinosis cutis, or tendon friction rubs should be evaluated for scleroderma (Varga, 2019). Varga (2019) presents that the initial diagnostic workup will likely include complete blood count that may reveal anemia, serum creatinine level that may indicate renal dysfunction, creatine kinase that may be elevated in the client with myopathy or myositis, and urinalysis that may reveal proteinuria and/or cellular casts. Although the skillful provider is aware that additional testing may include antinuclear antibody, antitopoisomerase I, antibody, anti-DNA topoisomerase I, anticentromere antibody, and anti-RNA polymerase III antibody, when the client is suspected to have scleroderma, a referral to a specialty provider is indicated. Some comorbid conditions that the primary care practitioner should be on alert for include Raynaud phenomenon (RP), heartburn and/or dysphagia of recent onset, characteristic nail fold capillary changes, erectile dysfunction in men, acute onset of hypertension and renal insufficiency, dyspnea on exertion, or diarrhea with malabsorption (Varga, 2019).

POLYMYALGIA RHEUMATICA

The older adult client who presents to the primary care setting with symmetrical aching and morning stiffness about the shoulders, hip girdle, torso, and neck that is worst on arising in the morning should be evaluated for polymyalgia rheumatica (Docken, 2020). A consult with a specialist may be prudent, as these symptoms resemble those that occur in a number of other immune or musculoskeletal conditions. Docken (2020) describes the typical lab findings of polymyalgia rheumatica as an elevated erythrocyte sedimentation rate and CRP, normocytic anemia, negative antinuclear antibodies, rheumatoid factor, cyclic citrullinated peptide antibodies, and normal creatine kinase. Symptom management includes low-dose glucocorticoids. Most clients will improve on 10 to 20 mg of prednisone per day after 3 days, with complete response within 3 weeks, and a lack of response strongly suggests the need for the provider to explore an alternative diagnosis (Docken, 2019).

Fast Facts

- The client who complains of symptoms of polyarthritis, typically affecting the hands and the feet, with morning stiffness or soreness reported, and systemic symptoms such as fatigue, weight loss, and low-grade fever for 6 weeks or more should be evaluated for rheumatoid arthritis.
- Live virus vaccines are contraindicated when symptoms of lupus are present or while the client is receiving immunosuppressive treatments (including prednisone).
- Patient education of the client with fatigue should be directed toward the incorporation of cognitive behavioral therapy, activity pacing, energy conservation, increasing physical activity, getting regular exercise, relaxation exercises, rest–activity balance, balanced diet, lifestyle moderation, stress management, time management, and sleep hygiene.
- Clients who present with dry eyes and dry mouth should be evaluated for Sjogren's syndrome.

(continued)

(continued)

- As gout is now considered to be a chronic inflammatory arthritis rather than an acute episodic condition, earlier initiation of urate-lowering therapies to prevent attacks is recommended.
- Interventions for psoriatic arthritis should be aimed at controlling inflammation and preventing discomfort, joint damage, and disability.
- Clients with fatigue, joint pain, puffy swollen fingers and/or nonpitting edema of the hands, skin thickening/tightening/ulcerations, abnormal nailfolds, cutaneous hyperpigmentation, calcinosis cutis, or tendon friction rubs should be evaluated for scleroderma.
- Most clients with polymyalgia rheumatica will improve on 10 to 20 mg of prednisone per day after 3 days, with complete response within 3 weeks, and a lack of response strongly suggests the need for the provider to explore an alternative diagnosis.

SUMMARY

This journey through the subspecialties continued with a collaborative clinical practice session with physician specialists and nurse practitioners practicing in specialty settings. Clients presented with common rheumatologic complaints that often begin with their visit to the primary care provider. This clinical immersion experience led to the identification of conditions that the primary care provider is expected to diagnose or perhaps initiate during the management of clients with musculoskeletal disease/variety of systemic autoimmune conditions. As always, effective management plans can only be developed once the provider has identified the correct etiology.

References

Baer, A. (2019). *Diagnosis and classification of Sjögren's syndrome.* UpToDate. Retrieved from https://www.uptodate.com/contents/diagnosis-and-classification-of-sjogrens-syndrome

Docken, W. (2019). *Treatment of polymyalgia rheumatica.* UpToDate. Retrieved from https://www.uptodate.com/contents/treatment-of-polymyalgia-rheumatica

Docken, W. (2020). *Clinical manifestations and diagnosis of polymyalgia rheumatica.* UpToDate. Retrieved from https://www.uptodate.com/contents/clinical-manifestations-and-diagnosis-of-polymyalgia-rheumatica

Gergianaki, I., & Bertsias, G. (2018). Systemic lupus erythematosus in primary care: An update and practical messages for the general practitioner. *Frontiers in Medicine (Lausanne), 5*, 161. doi:10.3389/fmed.2018.00161

Gladman, D., & Ritchlin, C. (2019). *Treatment of psoriatic arthritis.* UpToDate. Retrieved from https://www.uptodate.com/contents/treatment-of-psoriatic-arthritis

Goldberg, D. (2017). The primary care provider's role in diagnosing and treating rheumatoid arthritis. *Practical Pain Management, 17*(5). Retrieved from https://www.practicalpainmanagement.com/pain/myofascial/inflammatory-arthritis/primary-care-provider-role-diagnosing-treating-rheumatoid

Mallen, C., Davenport, G., Hui, M., Nuki, G., & Roddy, E. (2017). Improving management of gout in primary care: A new UK management guideline. *British Journal of General Practice, 67*(659), 284–285. doi:10.3399/bjgp17X691313

Sanicki, S., & Ozbalkan, Z. (2015). Fatigue in rheumatic diseases. *European Journal of Rheumatology, 2*(3), 109–113. doi:10.5152/eurjrheum.2015.0029

Varga, J. (2019). *Clinical manifestations and diagnosis of systemic sclerosis (scleroderma) in adults (2020).* UpToDate. Retrieved from https://www.uptodate.com/contents/clinical-manifestations-and-diagnosis-of-systemic-sclerosis-scleroderma-in-adults

Yu, D., & van Tubergen, A. (2019). *Clinical manifestations of axial spondyloarthritis (ankylosing spondylitis and nonradiographic axial spondyloarthritis) in adults.* UpToDate. Retrieved from https://www.uptodate.com/contents/clinical-manifestations-of-axial-spondyloarthritis-ankylosing-spondylitis-and-nonradiographic-axial-spondyloarthritis-in-adults

20

Practice Essentials for Urology

The adult client may present to primary care settings with a variety of symptoms related to the urological system. Although many of these conditions are appropriate for the primary care provider to diagnose and manage, some conditions may be emergent in nature or significant enough to be referred to the urologist or surgeon for management. The skillful provider is knowledgeable on the standards of care for the client with a urological condition, as well as the red flags to assess and refer for emergency care when indicated.

HEMATURIA

Clients may present to the primary care setting complaining of blood in the urine, or asymptomatic hematuria may be detected on urinalysis as part of a periodic health maintenance examination. Hematuria may also be present in those with high levels of calcium in the urine or those with inherited conditions, such as polycystic kidney disease, certain types of hemophilia, and sickle cell disease (National Kidney Foundation, n.d.). A comprehensive health history, complete physical examination, diagnostic workup, including laboratory testing (e.g., urinalysis and/or culture, as well as blood work for complete blood count, blood urea nitrogen/creatinine, electrolytes, and photothrombin/international normalized ratio/platelet count if taking anticoagulants) and imaging studies (e.g., ultrasound, kidney, ureter, and bladder [KUB], and/or CT scan), and consideration of referral to a specialist for consultation and further evaluation via cystoscopy are critical elements of the initial workup. Once identification of the correct condition is made, an effective management plan can be developed and implemented.

Microscopic hematuria may or may not be a significant finding. For instance, further investigation should be initiated in the case of the clients aged 40 years or older and/or the clients who smoke presenting with microscopic hematuria (Barkin, Rosenberg, & Miner, 2014). Adult clients who have microscopic hematuria with normal blood pressure and kidney function should have persistent microscopic hematuria evaluated via renal ultrasound, urine for protein, calcium, and creatinine, and blood testing for renal function, and adult hypertensive clients with abnormal blood tests, a family history of kidney disease, or high levels of protein in the urine should be referred for a renal biopsy (National Kidney Foundation, n.d.).

However, the skillful provider who evaluates the client who presents with macroscopic or "gross" hematuria must determine the pain status, where in the urinary stream the hematuria is noted, and if there are any blood clots present (Barkin et al., 2014). Barkin et al. (2014) describe some possible etiologies of gross hematuria with their corresponding recommendations for management (Table 20.1).

Table 20.1

Management of Gross Hematuria		
Type	**Description**	**Management**
Gross hematuria with unilateral pain	Usually represents renal colic suggesting patient is passing a ureteric stone on the affected side	Consider CT and referral
Gross hematuria throughout the stream with pelvic pain	Suggests hemorrhagic cystitis, acute bacterial prostatitis, a bladder tumor, or a bladder stone	Urine culture and CT/referral if negative culture
Gross hematuria and only pelvic pain	Suggests infection; a negative urine culture raises suspicion of bladder tumor	Urine culture and CT/referral if negative culture

Source: Data from Barkin, J., Rosenberg, M., & Miner, M. (2014). A guide to the management of urologic dilemmas for the primary care physician (PCP). *The Canadian Journal of Urology, 21*(Suppl. 2), 55–63.

Overall, the workup of the client who presents to the primary care setting with hematuria must take into account factors such as the age of the client, lifestyle behaviors, comorbid conditions, presence or absence of pain and other related symptoms, significance of the bleeding, and where in the stream the bleeding occurs. Due to the risk of pathology in the absence of infection, often a CT scan and/or referral to urology for cystoscopy/further management is appropriate.

CYSTITIS

Female clients who present to the primary care setting with a sudden onset of urinary frequency, urgency, and dysuria with or without hematuria, and without fever often related to sexual intercourse or prolonged retention of urine are typically diagnosed with simple cystitis (Barkin et al., 2014). With the first episode of cystitis, the female client is typically managed with a 3-day course of antibiotics. First-line agents for uncomplicated acute cystitis in the female client include nitrofurantoin monohydrate/macrocrystals, trimethoprim–sulfamethoxazole (TMP–SMX), or fosfomycin; β-lactam antibiotics may be used when other agents are not tolerated; fosfomycin and nitrofurantoin monohydrate/macrocrystals should be avoided when pyelonephritis is suspected; and fluoroquinolones should be reserved in the case of complicated cystitis (Brusch, 2020).

Barkin et al. (2014) add that in the event that a positive urine culture recurs more than two times a year, then a 10-day course of antibiotic therapy and a workup including a renal and pelvic ultrasound (KUB) is appropriate. If the preliminary diagnostic workup is abnormal or the female client has more than two episodes of cystitis in a year, fever, or an elevated white blood cell count, a referral to urology is indicated.

Fast Facts

Client education is the cornerstone of the management of cystitis. For instance, the female client should be instructed on lifestyle changes, such as wiping in the right direction, not holding her urine when she has the urge to void, double voiding, and voiding frequently and after intercourse; these lifestyle modifications may help prevent the recurrence of simple cystitis.

Finally, any man with a documented, urine culture-proven urinary tract infection should be referred to urology for evaluation and management (Barkin et al., 2014).

INTERSTITIAL CYSTITIS

Interstitial cystitis is a complex clinical syndrome. Clients may initially present to the primary care setting complaining of daytime and nighttime urinary frequency, urgency, and pelvic pain. As there is no clear etiology, pathophysiology, or clear diagnostic criteria, most often the primary care provider may not be able to devote the resources necessary for comprehensive evaluation and management. Universally effective treatments do not exist, so management consists of a combination of supportive, behavioral, and pharmacologic interventions (Rovner, 2018a). Interventions may include one or more of the following: oral pharmacologic agents (e.g., pentosan polysulfate sodium, antihistamines, tricyclic antidepressants, analgesics, antiinflammatory agents); intravesical therapy (e.g., medications intermittently instilled directly into the bladder via a catheter); surgical therapies; electrical stimulation; and/or complementary therapies (e.g., acupuncture, hypnosis, pelvic floor massage; Rovner, 2018b). A collaborative approach to management involving the primary care practitioner, urology, and a mental health specialist is often indicated in the treatment of clients with interstitial cystitis.

URINARY INCONTINENCE

Clients will initially present to the primary care setting with a complaint of involuntary urinary leakage. As there are a number of types of urinary incontinence, prior to the initiation of management, it is critical to determine the correct type. This section focuses on the more common types of urinary incontinence that will likely be identified, diagnosed, and/or managed by the primary care practitioner. Lukacz (2019) describes the various types of urinary incontinence with corresponding management recommendations, which are presented in Table 20.2.

Lifestyle modifications include the encouragement of weight loss; restriction of fluid intake before bedtime; minimal intake of caffeine and alcohol; smoking cessation; and incorporation of measures to reduce constipation. A trial of vaginal estrogen therapy may be useful for perimenopausal or postmenopausal women with either stress or urge incontinence. Stress incontinence may be managed using a variety of devices, duloxetine, or surgery, whereas urge incontinence can be treated with antimuscarinic agents, such as darifenacin, fesoterodine, oxybutynin, solifenacin, tolterodine, and trospium, or β-adrenergic therapy, such as mirabegron (Lukacz, 2019).

Table 20.2

Urinary Incontinence Management		
Type	Description	Management
Stress incontinence	Urine leaks with coughing, sneezing, laughing, exercising, or heavy lifting	■ Lifestyle modifications ■ Pelvic floor muscle exercise ■ Bladder training
Urge incontinence	A sudden, intense urge to urinate followed by an involuntary loss of urine; may include urinary frequency and nocturia	■ Lifestyle modifications ■ Pelvic floor muscle exercise ■ Bladder training is most effective for urge incontinence
Mixed incontinence	Experiencing more than one type of urinary incontinence	■ Lifestyle modifications ■ Pelvic floor muscle exercise ■ Bladder training

Source: Data from Lukacz, E. (2019). *Treatment of urinary incontinence in women*. UpToDate. Retrieved from https://www.uptodate.com/contents/treatment-of-urinary-incontinence-in-females

Clients who do not respond to first-line agents should typically be referred to an expert in urinary incontinence for evaluation and management.

FLANK PAIN

Nephrolithiasis

The client with renal colic will likely present to the primary care setting in severe pain, which initiates in the flank and back just under the ribs and radiates around the side and down onto the pelvis and testicles in a man or to the labia/vagina in a woman. The pain is typically accompanied by nausea, vomiting, and/or hematuria, and diagnosis of renal calculi is most often made following an ultrasound, a urinalysis, a plain KUB x-ray, and, if available, a CT scan. Prompt referral to a specialty provider is indicated (Barkin et al., 2014).

Pyelonephritis

The client who presents with fever, costovertebral angle pain, and nausea and/or vomiting, with or without the symptoms of cystitis and costovertebral angle tenderness, should be evaluated for pyelonephritis (Fulop, 2019a). The diagnostic workup for pyelonephritis includes urinalysis and urine culture, and imaging may be indicated in select client populations such as those with HIV/AIDS, poorly controlled diabetes, who have a history of renal transplant, other immunocompromised state, or sepsis (Fulop, 2019c).

Younger, nonpregnant women with uncomplicated acute pyelonephritis may be candidates for outpatient management, yet hospital admission should be considered in clients who are severely ill, pregnant, elderly, or who have comorbid disorders. Empiric therapy includes fluoroquinolones, cephalosporins, penicillins, extended-spectrum penicillins, carbapenems, and aminoglycosides (Fulop, 2019b).

CONDITIONS OF THE PROSTATE GLAND

Some conditions of the prostate gland are asymptomatic, and some male clients may present to primary care settings with symptoms related to the prostate gland. They may also present for health maintenance activities where prostate screening is indicated. Male clients aged 55 to 69 years should engage in shared decision-making with their primary care provider in order to make well-informed decisions about preventive services such as prostate cancer screening; men aged 70 years or older should not be screened for prostate cancer (American Academy of Family Physicians, 2018). Although professional groups do not all agree about the age to initiate periodic prostate cancer screening, the Canadian, American, and European Urological Associations all recommend regular screening for men over the age of 50 years (Barkin et al., 2014). Abnormalities of the prostate gland must be evaluated by a specialist with expertise in urological conditions, such as pathology of the prostate gland. Blood testing, diagnostic imaging, and/or biopsy of the prostate gland may be part of the evaluation of disorders of the prostate.

It has been reported that the total prostate-specific antigen (PSA) test has a 75% sensitivity, but only a 40% specificity, for detecting prostate cancer as it is produced by both benign and malignant cells (Barkin et al., 2014).

Fast Facts

Although normal values vary depending on client's age and race, a PSA of ≥4 ng/mL is widely accepted as indicating a suspicion of prostate cancer in men who are 60 years and older, and according to Barkin et al. (2014), serum PSA may be elevated in clients with the following conditions:

(continued)

(continued)

- Prostatitis or urinary tract infection: Those who have had recent sexual activity or significant bike riding
- Significant benign prostatic hyperplasia (BPH): Those who have had a vigorous digital rectal examination
- Prostate cancer: Those who have undergone recent urethral instrumentation

Clients with elevated PSA should be referred to urology for consultation to determine whether a biopsy is indicated to rule out prostate cancer.

Acute Bacterial Prostatitis

Prostatitis syndromes tend to occur in young and middle-aged male clients. Although clients who have undergone recent prostate biopsy or those who are HIV infected may be at higher risk, most clients with acute bacterial prostatitis have no clear risk factors. Meyrier and Fekete (2019) describe that the client may present acutely ill, with fever, chills, malaise, myalgia, dysuria, frequency, urgency, urge incontinence, dribbling, poor stream, hesitancy, cloudy urine, and pain in the pelvic or perineal regions and/or at the tip of the penis. On exam, the prostate is typically firm, edematous, and tender. As acute bacterial prostatitis is most typically caused by gram-negative organisms, antimicrobial therapy remains the mainstay of treatment (Meyrier & Fekete, 2019).

Possible complications of acute bacterial prostatitis include bacteremia, epididymitis, chronic bacterial prostatitis, prostatic abscesses, and metastatic infection, so a urine Gram stain and culture should be obtained in clients suspected of having acute prostatitis (Meyrier & Fekete, 2019). Imaging studies are generally not indicated, unless there is suspicion of prostatic abscess. The client with recurrent infections should consult with urology.

Management recommendations include TMP–SMX (one double-strength tablet every 12 hours) or a fluoroquinolone (ciprofloxacin 500 mg every 12 hours or levofloxacin 500 mg once daily) as empiric therapy. A 28-day course of therapy is indicated (Meyrier & Fekete, 2019). Men younger than 35 years who are sexually active and men older than 35 years who engage in high-risk sexual behavior should be treated to cover *Neisseria gonorrhoeae* and *Chlamydia trachomatis*, and those with persistently positive urine cultures should be further evaluated and treated for chronic bacterial prostatitis (Meyrier & Fekete, 2019).

Benign Prostatic Hypertrophy

The adult and older adult male clients with benign prostatic hypertrophy may present to the primary care setting complaining of symptoms of increased frequency of urination, nocturia, hesitancy, urgency, and weak urinary stream (Cunningham & Kadmon, 2019).

Fast Facts

The client without discomfort or complication (e.g., bladder outlet obstruction, renal insufficiency, or recurrent infection) may not require pharmacologic management, benefiting from behavioral modifications as follows:

- Avoiding fluids prior to bedtime
- Limiting fluids before going out
- Reducing consumption of mild diuretics, such as caffeine
- Minimizing intake of alcohol
- Double voiding to empty the bladder more completely
- Avoiding medications that may exacerbate symptoms, such as diuretics
- Discontinuing medications that may induce retention, such as an opioid or antipsychotic medication

Evidence suggests that clients with BPH require therapy only if symptoms have a significant impact on quality of life or they develop complications, such as hydronephrosis, renal insufficiency, urinary retention, recurrent infection, or bladder decompensation (Cunningham & Kadmon, 2019). A referral to a urologist is indicated in clients who have recently underwent an invasive treatment of the urethra or prostate, are over age of 45 years, have an abnormality on prostate exam, demonstrate hematuria or incontinence, or report severe symptoms. In patients with mild-to-moderate symptoms, initial treatment is with an α1-adrenergic antagonist, such as terazosin, doxazosin, tamsulosin, alfuzosin, or silodosin; however, a 5α-reductase inhibitor, such as finasteride or dutasteride, is also an alternative in patients who do not tolerate the first-line therapies (Cunningham & Kadmon, 2019).

ERECTILE DYSFUNCTION

The male client may first report symptoms of erectile dysfunction to the primary care provider. The initial workup includes a comprehensive medical, sexual, and psychosocial history along with a focused physical examination and select diagnostic testing, such as serum total testosterone levels. Comorbid conditions known to affect erectile dysfunction, such as diabetes, heart disease, or depression, must be addressed. Lifestyle modifications, such as changes in diet and increased activity levels, are to be encouraged. Initial medical management should include sildenafil, tadalafil, vardenafil, or avanafil (Mayo Clinic, 2018a). The client may be referred to consult with a mental health professional and/or urology for persistent symptoms, as additional diagnostic evaluation such as an ultrasound of the penis should be considered and additional therapeutic options such as a vacuum erection device or intracavernosal injections presented (Burnett et al., 2018).

UROLOGIC EMERGENCIES

At times, clients will present to primary care settings for care of a condition of the urinary system, which may be emergent in nature. It is the role of the seasoned primary care practitioner to provide a thorough assessment and determine a preliminary diagnosis/management plan. Often in the primary care setting, it is critical for the provider to decide whether an emergency consultation with urology or a surgeon should be indicated.

Paraphimosis

When the male client presents to the primary care setting with conditions such as the foreskin retracted behind the head of the penis, tightness of the foreskin, and some swelling of the glans, causing the inability to bring the foreskin back over the head of the penis, a diagnosis of paraphimosis is likely (Barkin et al., 2014). Due to the risk of strangulation of the head of the penis and necrosis, the presenting condition could be emergent in nature. Ice may be used temporarily to decrease the swelling and numb the discomfort while an emergency evaluation with a specialist is arranged (Barkin et al., 2014).

Hernia

The male client may present to the primary care setting complaining of a bulge in the inguinal region that may or may not be tender, transilluminate, or able to be reduced. Often, these symptoms that likely indicate an inguinal hernia initiate after heavy lifting. As an incarcerated, painful hernia is a surgical emergency, a referral to a surgeon is indicated (Barkin et al., 2014).

Adult Hydrocele

The adult male client may also present to the primary care setting with a chief complaint of scrotal edema. Hydroceles, or fluid surrounding one or both testicles, may occur as a result of a traumatic injury, inflammation, or infection and typically do not require urgent treatment. However, a hydrocele that develops as a reaction to a testicular tumor must be treated urgently by removing the tumor and so prompt referral to a specialist for proper diagnosis and management is indicated (Barkin et al., 2014).

Testicular Pain

The young adult male client may present to the primary care setting with testicular pain, often waking him in the middle of the night. The testicle is tender upon assessment, and there may be significant scrotal edema noted. These suggest the likelihood of a testicular torsion, an acute emergency condition. As there is only about a 6-hour window from the time of pain onset until an emergency repair to salvage the testicle, an emergent referral is indicated (Barkin et al., 2014).

Another condition to consider in the client who presents complaining of testicular pain in the presence of swelling, fever, nausea, vomiting, and malaise that can be secondary to heavy lifting, a bowel movement, or even sexual activity may indicate orchitis, or an inflammation of one or both testicles (Mayo Clinic, 2018b). Bacterial or viral infections (e.g., mumps) can cause orchitis, or the cause can be unknown. As orchitis is most often the result of a bacterial infection, such as a sexually transmitted infection, the skillful provider takes this factor into account while gathering the client's history and determining the management plan (Barkin et al., 2014). As infertility is a possible complication of orchitis, prompt management and consultation with a specialty provider may be considered while planning care.

Overall, the primary care provider must include education on primary prevention strategies, which include testicular health. Male clients should be instructed to perform monthly self-examination of testicles. Prompt medical attention should be sought in the event a hard, nontender lump is detected (Barkin et al., 2014).

RENAL CYST

The seasoned primary care provider is aware that although most renal cysts are found incidentally and asymptomatic, they occasionally become large enough to cause pain, hematuria, hypertension, or obstruction (Bas et al., 2015). Others can be suspicious for malignancy. Once apparent, renal cysts should be monitored as per published guidelines, such as the Bosniak classification system of renal cystic masses described in Table 20.3.

Table 20.3

Bosniak Classification of Renal Cystic Masses	
Category I	Benign simple renal cyst or multiple renal cysts, each with a thin wall without septa, calcifications, or solid components
Category II	Benign cystic lesions in which there may be a few thin septa, and the wall or septa may contain fine calcifications or a short segment of slightly thickened calcification; uniformly high-attenuation lesions that are <3 cm in diameter, well margined, and nonenhancing
Category IIF	Well margined and are more complicated cysts than category II cysts but less complicated than category III cysts, which may have multiple thin septa or minimal smooth thickening of the septa or wall and contain calcification; may also be thick and nodular; no measurable contrast enhancement; includes totally intrarenal, nonenhancing, high-attenuating lesions that are >3 cm in diameter; require follow-up to evaluate for malignancy
Category III	Indeterminate cystic masses that have thickened, irregular or smooth walls or septa; measurable enhancement is present; 40% to 60% malignant (cystic renal cell carcinoma and multiloculated cystic renal cell carcinoma); referral indicated; remaining lesions are benign, such as hemorrhagic cysts, chronic infected cysts, or nephroma
Category IV	Have all the characteristics of category III cysts, plus contain enhancing soft tissue components that are adjacent to and independent of the wall or septum; 85% to 100% malignant; referral indicated

Source: Data from Silverman, S. G., Pedrosa, I., Ellis, J. H., Hindman, N. H., Schieda, N., Smith, A. D., & Davenport, M. S. (2019). *Bosniak classification of cystic renal masses, version 2019: An update proposal and needs assessment.* Retrieved from https://pubs.rsna.org/doi/10.1148/radiol.2019182646

- Due to the risk of pathology with gross hematuria in the absence of infection, often a CT scan and/or referral to urology for cystoscopy/further management is appropriate.
- In the event that a positive urine culture recurs more than two times a year in the client with cystitis, then a 10-day course of antibiotic therapy and a workup including a renal and pelvic ultrasound (KUB) is appropriate.
- As there is no clear etiology, pathophysiology, or clear diagnostic criteria, most often the primary care provider may not be able to devote the resources necessary for comprehensive evaluation and management of interstitial cystitis.
- Lifestyle modifications to manage urinary incontinence include the encouragement of weight loss; restriction of fluid intake before bedtime; minimal intake of alcohol or caffeine; smoking cessation; and measures to reduce constipation.
- Prompt referral to a specialty provider is indicated in emergent urological conditions.
- Clients with BPH require therapy only if symptoms have a significant impact on quality of life or they develop complications.
- The initial workup of erectile dysfunction includes a comprehensive medical, sexual, and psychosocial history along with a focused physical examination and select diagnostic testing, such as serum total testosterone levels.
- Renal cysts should be monitored as per the Bosniak classification system of renal cystic masses.

SUMMARY

This journey through the subspecialties continued with a collaborative clinical practice session with physician specialists and nurse practitioners practicing in specialty settings. Clients presented with common urological complaints that often begin with their visit to the primary care provider. This clinical immersion experience led to the identification of conditions that the primary care provider is expected to diagnose or perhaps initiate during the management of clients with a variety of conditions affecting the urological system. As always, effective management plans can only be developed once the provider has identified the correct etiology.

References

American Academy of Family Physicians. (2018). *AAFP updates its PSA screening recommendation.* Retrieved from https://www.aafp.org/news/health-of-the-public/20180720aafppsarec.html

Barkin, J., Rosenberg, M., & Miner, M. (2014). A guide to the management of urologic dilemmas for the primary care physician (PCP). *The Canadian Journal of Urology, 21*(Suppl. 2), 55–63.

Bas, O., Nalbant, I., Can Sener, N., Firat, H., Yeşil, S., Zengin, K., & Imamoglu, A. (2015). Management of renal cysts. *Journal of the Society of Laparoendoscopic Surgeons, 19*(1), e2014.00097. doi:10.4293/JSLS.2014.00097

Brusch, J. L. (2020). *Urinary tract infection (UTI) and cystitis (bladder infection) in females treatment & management.* Retrieved from https://emedicine.medscape.com/article/233101-treatment

Burnett, A. L., Nehra, A., Breau, R. H., Culkin, D. J., Faraday, M. M., Hakim, L. S., & Shindel, A. W. (2018). *Erectile dysfunction: AUA guideline (2018).* Retrieved from https://www.auanet.org/guidelines/erectile-dysfunction-(ed)-guideline

Cunningham, G., & Kadmon, D. (2019). *Medical treatment of benign prostatic hyperplasia.* UpToDate. Retrieved from https://www.uptodate.com/contents/medical-treatment-of-benign-prostatic-hyperplasia

Fulop, T. (2019a). *Acute pyelonephritis clinical presentation.* Retrieved from https://emedicine.medscape.com/article/245559-clinical

Fulop, T. (2019b). *Acute pyelonephritis treatment & management.* Retrieved from https://emedicine.medscape.com/article/245559-treatment

Fulop, T. (2019c). *Acute pyelonephritis workup.* Retrieved from https://emedicine.medscape.com/article/245559-workup#c10

Lukacz, E. (2019). *Treatment of urinary incontinence in women.* UpToDate. Retrieved from https://www.uptodate.com/contents/treatment-of-urinary-incontinence-in-females

Mayo Clinic. (2018a). *Erectile dysfunction.* Retrieved from https://www.mayoclinic.org/diseases-conditions/erectile-dysfunction/diagnosis-treatment/drc-20355782

Mayo Clinic. (2018b). *Orchitis.* Retrieved from https://www.mayoclinic.org/diseases-conditions/orchitis/symptoms-causes/syc-20375860

Meyrier, A., & Fekete, T. (2019). *Acute bacterial prostatitis.* UpToDate. Retrieved from https://www.uptodate.com/contents/acute-bacterial-prostatitis

National Kidney Foundation. (n.d.). *Hematuria in adults.* Retrieved from https://www.kidney.org/atoz/content/hematuria-adults

Rovner, E. S. (2018a). *Interstitial cystitis.* Retrieved from https://emedicine.medscape.com/article/2055505-overview

Rovner, E. S. (2018b). *Interstitial cystitis treatment & management.* Retrieved from https://emedicine.medscape.com/article/2055505-treatment

Silverman, S. G., Pedrosa, I., Ellis, J. H., Hindman, N. H., Schieda, N., Smith, A. D., & Davenport, M. S. (2019). *Bosniak classification of cystic renal masses, version 2019: An update proposal and needs assessment.* Retrieved from https://pubs.rsna.org/doi/10.1148/radiol.2019182646

Index

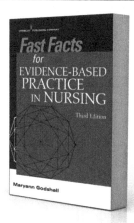
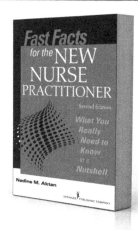
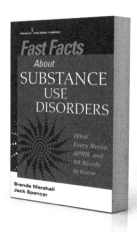
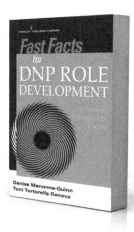

Printed in the United States
by Baker & Taylor Publisher Services